LIFE IN THE A-ZONE

How I embraced the journey with

my mother's Alzheimer's

one pink cloud moment at a time

Peggy Sweeney-McDonald

Life in the A-Zone

Copyright © 2025 by Peggy Sweeney-McDonald

Published by
Pink Cloud Publishing
Baton Rouge, Louisiana

First Edition: 2025

ISBN: 979-8-9994729-0-8 (Paperback)
ISBN: 979-8-9994729-2-2 (eBook)
ISBN: 979-8-9994729-3-9 (Audiobook)

Printed in the United States of America

For information, visit:
www.lifeinthea-zone.com
www.peggysweeneymcdonald.com

For my beloved mother,

Sherry Murphy Sweeney

who taught me how to love, laugh, and look for

pink cloud moments every day.

TABLE OF CONTENTS

EARLY PRAISE FOR LIFE IN THE A-ZONE

Life in the A-Zone brought tears to my eyes with its delicate and soulful touch. As I turned the pages, it gently nudged me to confront the long-ignored grief of my mother's battle with Alzheimer's—a journey I hadn't fully faced, especially after the tragic loss of my daughter. This book arrived as a quiet gift, guiding me back through that hard and audacious road with grace, compassion, and recognition. This book is for anyone who has lost, loved, and longed to feel seen again. It felt like it saw me.
— Karen McCord, Author of *Only Rainbows: The Carley McCord Story*

This is a moving and deeply human story of love, caregiving, and resilience, set against the rich backdrop of Louisiana's culture, cuisine, and heart. It draws you in from the first page!
— *Jax Frey,* Author of *The Gumbeaux Sistahs novels*

Peggy Sweeney-McDonald stirs together the savory and the not-so-savory ingredients that make up the gumbo of life when caring for an Alzheimer's patient, in this case, Peggy's mother. You feel the pain and sadness, but you also get the beautiful, one-of-a-kind moments that are part of this journey. And to make it even more special, Peggy ladles in some of the South Louisiana recipes that give her story deeper meaning and a sense of place.
— Paul Wilborn, Author of *Florida Hustle and Cigar City*

Through her vulnerable storytelling and true-to-life candor, Peggy shines light on the entire 'family journey' through the dis-ease of Alzheimer's. The stories honor the honest truths while creating space for the kindred community of so many souls who have trudged—and are trudging—the caregiver's journey.
— Amanda Rieger Green, MPH, Host of *Soul Pathology Podcast*

Every chapter in *Life in the A-Zone* is a pink cloud moment waiting to be felt. Peggy captures the dance of grief and grace with the kind of hope only someone who's lived it can give.
— Sabrina Johnson, MDiv, Author of *How to Sit & Stay with Compassionate Meditation*, and Host of *Listen Up Listen In* Podcast

Peggy has offered her readers a poignant and moving story of how a Louisiana family deals with the challenge of Alzheimer's. She also expressively shares her vast knowledge of food and recipes from the Bayou State—an emotional saga of living a challenging life.
— Jim Brown, Publisher, The Lisburn Press

Life in the A-Zone is like sitting with Peggy on a veranda in rocking chairs, sipping iced tea while listening to her tell her stories. The pain and sadness are there among all the textures, colors, sounds, and tastes of life as she was experiencing her journey with her mother's Alzheimer's. This book is a love letter to anyone who has walked a parent home. Peggy's storytelling is a gift.
— Maxine Crump, Executive Director, Dialogue on Race Louisiana

An authentic and vulnerable journey about caring for a parent with Alzheimer's.
— Jean Trebek, Co-Founder/Podcast Co-Host, *InsideWink*

Life in the A-Zone is an essential read for anyone navigating a similar path, or for those who simply wish to understand the human heart in its most vulnerable state. It is a story told with immense heart and an unforgettable voice.
— Jennifer Fink, Host of *Fading Memories* Podcast

"I'm back."
"From where?"
From an amazing respite, a renewing journey into the world of *Life in the A-Zone*. Peggy Sweeney-McDonald's tender storytelling spoke to my soul, soothing both my eyes and my heart. Her words afforded me the opportunity—and provided the vehicle—to briefly slip away from my role as caregiver and to exhale, drop my shoulders, breathe, and simply be. Thank you, Peggy, for this beautiful and healing work.
—Jay Westbrook, author of *Compassionate Journeys: Lessons From My Work With The Dying* and Clinical Director of Grief Recovery of Tupelo

Peggy draws readers in with a heartfelt and immersive narrative, making them feel as though they are walking alongside her through a deeply personal journey. Her story—painful, raw, and moving—captures the enduring love between a mother and daughter as they navigate the heartbreaking realities of Alzheimer's. A powerful testament to family, resilience, and compassion. This is a must-read for anyone seeking understanding and hope in the face of loss.
— Gisele Harrison, Author, *Who Says You Can't, A Workbook to Success*

Peggy captures the emotional complexity of caregiving—the grief, the love, the fatigue, and even unexpected beauty. Her story is deeply personal yet universal, offering hope and connection to anyone navigating this journey.
— Pennie Nichols, Author and Retreat Facilitator

What a gift this book is! Peggy doesn't just tell us her story—she invites us into the quiet heartbreak and sacred resilience of caregiving. You'll cry, nod your head, and feel seen in every chapter."
— Victoria Greene, Director/Producer of *Forgotten Bayou*

Beautiful, poignant memories of a daddy's girl navigating the waters of her mother's Alzheimer's. Narrated with heart and soul, Peggy takes us on a journey of reaffirmation of a dynamic love between dynamic women. Thank you, Peggy, for a view from the box seats.
— Stephaun Paul, Actor

As a psychotherapist sitting with caregivers dealing with a loved one afflicted with Alzheimer's or other dementias, I witness firsthand the utter devastation and bottomless pit of powerlessness this disease inflicts on all connected to it. I also experienced it personally with my own mother. *Life in the A-Zone* offers up to us a generous banquet of community and healing, and the exquisite felt sense that even during such painful grief and loss it truly is small moments of love and grace that matter most meaningfully in the end.
— Sherry Stuart Berman, Psychotherapist and Poet

INTRODUCTION

Can you imagine if we could take all the caregiving stories and share them with people who have just begun the "A-Zone" with their loved ones, as I named the journey with my mother's Alzheimer's? Would it make a difference to know in advance the hardship, the struggle, the tears, the anger, the pain, and the heartbreak that would come along with caregiving? Would it make a difference to know that, in the turbulence of caregiving, there can be moments when you can smile, laugh, hug, kiss, hold hands with your loved one, and recall the good times? Those pink cloud moments are moments of grace, and they can heal your heart in the toughest of times. These moments will live on in your heart even after your loved one is gone, and you will be blessed for having discovered and remembered them.

It has been six years since my mother passed away. Each year gets a little easier. I cling to the good memories of when she was healthy and full of life. Still, I remember the day she was officially diagnosed in vivid detail—the day the rug was pulled out from under us, the day that our family began trudging the A-Zone without a road map. I knew at that moment my life would change forever. By divine intervention, my husband, Jimmy, was laid off that same afternoon from his job as a stockbroker. Within months, we sold our condo in Los Angeles, drove across the country, and moved in with my parents to Baton Rouge, Louisiana. It was heartbreaking, gut-wrenching, and the most challenging three years of my life. Yet there were beautiful lessons of love, laughter, life, and loss while living in the A-Zone. I learned to find gratitude in the little victories every day, to dig deep for courage, and to rely on my higher power as I became my mother's caregiver.

With no children of my own, I was not equipped to be a caregiver. I struggled emotionally, watching my beautiful and vibrant mother slip away before my eyes. "Come back, please," I wanted to scream every day.

My mother passed away on July 2, 2019. I was grateful she was no longer suffering. However, I wasn't prepared for the grief, the guilt, and the emptiness. There were so many things I could have done differently. I regretted moving away 36 years before and missing her good years. I regretted the times I wasn't patient and lost my temper. I wanted one more day with her, even if it was one of the bad days.

As I walked around the beautiful lake in our neighborhood, the still small voice inside me—which I thought was my intuition, but now believe was my mother, my angel, whispered to me to write my stories. With the rising number of people across the world affected by Alzheimer's, I knew each one had family members trudging through the caregiving struggle. I may not be able to create a cure for the disease, but I could share my experience, strength, and hope. Perhaps my stories could help another caregiver realize they aren't alone in the Alzheimer's battle.

For months, I stared at my laptop every day. *I should begin writing*, I told myself, but I had a list of reasons not to start. Instead, I chose to nap, exercise, cook, eat, or binge-watch a streaming show. Then I saw the 2019 Louisiana Book Festival schedule offering a memoir essay writing class, and I felt the nudge to register. This class could jump-start my writing. On a crisp November day, I walked into the class, dressed up in my favorite leggings with black boots, a fall sweater, my leather jacket, and a hat. With makeup on, including bright pink lipstick, I felt cute, motivated, and alive that morning.

Following a writing prompt given by the instructor, I wrote my first story, The Fashion Show. In it, I shared my feelings about watching my mother—a proper southern woman always dressed fashionably—reduced by Alzheimer's to dressing in mismatched, inside-out, and sometimes dirty clothes. When I read my story to the class, my voice broke, and I began to cry. Looking up, I found the instructor and the other participants crying too. The instructor looked at me and said, "You just wrote that?" I nodded. She replied, "You must write your story, Peggy. You will help many people going through the same thing."

Walking out of the class, I felt lighter and inspired. I now had a purpose. I soon began going to the local CC's Coffee House with my laptop. I wrote with passion and urgency I had never known before. I would grab a coffee, sit down, and start. Hours passed quickly; my coffee grew cold and untouched. The stories poured out of my heart, and I felt my mother guiding me. I didn't write them in any order. A story would pop up, and I would begin.

Hours later, I would come home, prepare dinner, and then read the story to my father and husband at the table. I'd look up to see tears in their eyes—or hear them laugh with me. My dad never cried when my mother passed away, but now the flood gates had opened. He no longer had to be the strong southern gentleman—he could be vulnerable and feel his feelings. We all healed sitting around the dinner table while my mother was watching over us.

As my memoir unfolded on the page, more life changes happened. My 84-year-old father had a knee replacement, I had a hysterectomy, and the pandemic began. I knew the book journey would be long and tedious. My first book, *Meanwhile, Back at Cafe Du Monde… Life Stories About Food*, by Pelican Publishing, was released in 2012 after years of work and a four-month book tour. I wasn't ready for queries, rejections, and the waiting game. I didn't want to wait for someone else to decide my stories were worth reading. I knew they were because they came from my heart with my mother's gentle nudging from above.

Soon, I heard "Get these stories out now," and I felt my mom was kicking me into action. On July 2, 2020—amid the COVID-19 pandemic—I met for a socially distanced visit with my two girlfriends, Jackie and Pennie, and told them I was thinking of sharing my stories in a podcast. They encouraged me, and on my birthday three weeks later, I booked studio time and recorded the first three episodes. On July 29th, I launched my *Life in the A-Zone* podcast. Within weeks, I had listeners around the world commenting on how my stories made them laugh and cry.

One of my oldest girlfriends, Nancy, is a voice-over actress, and she taught me over Zoom how to record and edit audio files in my make-shift studio, a walk-in closet. I found a gifted sound engineer, Slavi, in Bulgaria, who added music and sound effects. Over the next six months, I recorded 20 episodes, beginning when my mother was diagnosed with Alzheimer's, and ending when she passed away. The podcast became an incredible, creative journey that lifted me out of depression and into healing action.

It has been five years since I created the podcast and shared my stories. I have long wanted to publish this book, and now my intuition is telling me that now is the time—to share it with the caregivers at the beginning, the middle, or end of the A-Zone, and those who are now on the other side.

These stories are the gift of coming home, the gift of being there for my mother, dad, and family. I believe my mother is smiling down, her spirit now among the other angels who also endured Alzheimer's, dementia, cancer, or any other life-threatening disease. Through the tough times, family caregivers are learning compassion, courage, hope, and strength. They are my heroes.

In reading this book, I hope you find a glimmer of hope within the pages. I hope you find the courage to take it a day at a time. And, in the hardest of days, I hope you find your pink cloud moments. And remember, love always wins. You are my hero!

CHAPTER ONE
THE DECISION

"Peanuts or pretzels?" the perky flight attendant asks me.

"Can I please have both?"

She hands me the mini snack packs, smiling, then gives me a bonus pack of peanuts—three for one. Ask, and you shall receive.

Today is a "more-is-more" snack day. It's only 10:00 a.m., but I open all the mini packs of snacks to go with my airplane coffee, which sucks, so I wash the salty snacks with my pricey bottled water purchased at the airport store. I reach for my equally costly gossip magazine and settle in for the four-hour flight to New Orleans. It has only been thirty minutes since take-off, but I need an emotional distraction. Reading about Hollywood stars getting divorced, starting a cooking show, and winning acting awards distracts my restless mind. I need gossip trash just like I need snack trash.

My vacation is wrought with dread. For the first time in years, I'm not excited to fly back "home" to Louisiana from my current home in Los Angeles. It's been six months since I was in Baton Rouge when we threw a big birthday brunch for my parents to celebrate Mom's 79th and Dad's 80th birthdays. The event was festive, with a catered brunch of shrimp and grits, a giant birthday cake, and a jazz band. I have never seen my parents happier, surrounded by their family and friends.

This two-week stay will include a weekend wedding in Alabama for my cousin, followed by Easter weekend, but most important is the neurologist appointment for my mother, who we agree probably has Alzheimer's. My sister, Shannan, decided we should all be there—my father and mother with all four daughters.

Shannan is an attorney, the second daughter, born 17 months after me. However, she has always been the "older sister," taking charge of everything. I may be the oldest on paper, but I was the creative one, the actress who left Baton Rouge in 1980 after graduating from Louisiana State University to pursue big dreams in Houston, New York, New Orleans, and finally settling in Los Angeles for the last 19 years. I had silently relinquished the "older daughter" baton years ago, and now, 36 years later, I'm filled with guilt for not having been there, especially these last challenging years. I'm happy to do whatever is asked of me now.

A wall of humidity hits me as I step out of the airport. It feels like summer. I'm hot and sticky within minutes, and my makeup is sliding down my cheeks. Welcome back to Louisiana!

Standing at the curb, I spot my parents and wave. My mother and father soon pull up next to me in their brown "Grandparents Van." Dad gets out, gives me a big bear hug, opens the hatch, and lifts my suitcase into the back. I am more than capable of raising my bag, but my 80-year-old father is the quintessential Southern gentleman and loves doing anything to help his girls and grandchildren. I jump into the backseat and lean over to kiss my mother. She is smiling and happy to see me.

"There's some bottled water in the ice chest by your feet. Are you hungry? I thought we would go eat at Harbor Seafood," Dad announces.

My father is always ready to feed and water us.

"Sounds great to me! All I've had to eat today was an apple, a cheese stick, and the freebie peanuts and pretzels."

Dad pulls out of the airport and heads to the restaurant in the New Orleans suburb of Kenner, or "Kennah," as everyone here calls it. Coming here has been a Sweeney tradition forever. My late grandparents lived nearby and loved their oyster poboys. Whenever Sweeney family members fly in or out of New Orleans airport, we make a stop at Harbor Seafood for a delicious meal before heading back to Baton Rouge.

It's two o'clock when we turn off Williams Boulevard, and I notice there isn't anyone waiting outside on the park bench or standing outside the door. We missed the lunch rush. Usually, you must wait outside for lunch at this popular spot. There are no parking spots in the front, so we drove back to park in the oyster shell parking lot. If you aren't from Louisiana, you probably won't know that we often use broken oyster shells instead of gravel for parking lots and driveways. At the sound of the oyster shells crunching under the tires, I know we have arrived at Harbor, and my mouth starts watering for their delicious seafood.

"Dad, don't forget to lock the van!" The thought of my suitcase getting stolen freaks me out. Never mind that I have a closet full of clothes in the guest room I use at my parents' home. My suitcase, stolen from a car trunk in New York City years ago, has left me with lasting paranoia. As

14

we enter the restaurant, I wonder if I'm putting it out into the universe for it to happen again or if my intuition is telling me, it will happen today. Maybe I'm just anxious about this trip. I tell myself to stop it and enjoy my parents. I need to be present. *Breathe, Peggy, breathe!*

The delicious smell of fried seafood and rich gumbo envelops us the minute we step through the door. It's the "real deal," as my husband, Jimmy, calls this intoxicating scent. Years ago, we were in Phoenix heading for a day trip to Sedona when I saw the big Pappadeaux's Seafood restaurant sign on the side of the freeway.

"Oh my God, there's a Pappadeaux's here!" I exclaimed.

"What the hell is Pappadeaux's?" Jimmy asked.

"It was my favorite Louisiana restaurant when I lived in Houston in the '80s."

I made a note of the exit, and later, returning from Sedona, we stopped for dinner. As soon as we entered Pappadeaux's, the smell of gumbo and fried seafood filled our nostrils. Jimmy turned to me and said, "It smells like the real deal." Soon, slurping a spoon of seafood gumbo, he said, "Yeah, you're right... the real deal!" For my New Yorker husband, loving Louisiana food was his coveted prize for marrying a southern girl.

I know Jimmy will be jealous that we are eating here. We follow the hostess to a table by the window, and a friendly waitress soon arrives, setting down giant plastic tumblers of iced water.

"How are y'all doing? My name is Sandy. What can I getcha to drink today, darlings?"

After giving Sandy our drink orders, we dug into the basket of individually wrapped saltine crackers with small foil packs of butter. I peruse the extensive menu. What to order?

Living in Los Angeles, I never get "real deal" seafood. I could eat it all: gumbo, crawfish etouffee, raw and charbroiled oysters, boiled seafood, fried seafood platters, crawfish pasta, poboys, and more. But here at Harbor Seafood, I always get the same thing: a cup of gumbo and the seafood-stuffed mirliton that comes with a side salad swimming in ranch dressing with a slice of buttered Texas toast. Dad orders gumbo and the seafood pasta special, and Mom wants a fried shrimp plate. Let the two-week Louisiana food fest begin! There is nothing like this in Los Angeles.

As we wait for our lunch, Dad excitedly tells me about the itinerary for the upcoming wedding weekend in Dauphin Island, Alabama. My sister, Erin, will join us. We will leave on Friday morning. It will be a fun road trip. Besides attending the rehearsal dinner and wedding, we will go to Bellingrath Gardens on Saturday and visit old friends on Sunday.

"Who's getting married?" Mom asks.

"Michael," Dad replies.

"Who's that?" she says. Dad explains it is his nephew: his late sister, Althea's son.

"Oh, that's right. How's your husband?" she asks me, forgetting Jimmy's name.

"Jimmy's fine. He misses his Mustang Convertible."

"What happened to it?" she asks. She had forgotten that Jimmy had been in a car accident last month.

"Some idiot pulled out of a parking lot and t-boned his baby. He wasn't hurt, but a boring Toyota Corolla has replaced the midlife crisis car he had driven for ten years. He will never be the same," I explain, and they laugh.

Sandy brings our seafood gumbo, and we dive into our bowls. Our table is covered with plastic and foil wrappers with cracker crumbs scattered over the red plastic tablecloth. Mom takes a bite of Dad's gumbo and eats more crackers. Dad and I inhaled our gumbo in minutes. The dark roux is delicious, and the bowl is brimming with oysters, shrimp, and crabmeat, with half of a crab hanging out of my bowl. After finishing the gumbo, I crack the crab shell with my knife, pick out the sweet crabmeat, and then suck out the juices from the crab claws. I leave nothing but the empty crab shell in the bowl. I'm in gumbo heaven until our entrees arrive.

"I didn't order this," Mom announces when Sandy delivers our entrees.

Dad and I look at each other. *What the ...?*

"Sherry, that's what you ordered," Dad states emphatically.

"No, I ordered that!" she proclaims, pointing to my plate.

Dad's face gets bright red as he rolls his eyes and continues arguing with her, making her even more upset.

"It's okay, Mom. We can split mine. I can't eat all of this anyway," I interrupt them while cutting my stuffed mirliton in half and placing it on her plate. She smiles at me and begins eating. I scoop a bunch of her fried shrimp and fries onto my plate. I squeeze lemon on everything and add hot sauce to the cocktail sauce, as it's never spicy enough for me. I dip the fried shrimp in the cocktail sauce and then into the homemade tartar sauce. It's melt-in-your-mouth delicious.

We eat in silence. Mom picks at her food. Damn, her memory loss is getting real! I'm ready for this meal to be over.

The ride "home" to Baton Rouge is an easy hour and fifteen minutes. Mom quickly falls asleep, and Dad has the Sirius radio '50s station playing, so he can't hear me talk from the backseat.

Jealous? Eat your heart out! I texted Jimmy, sending him a picture of my yummy seafood lunch.

You are mean. I hope you aren't going to do this for the next two weeks! He texted back.

We pulled into the driveway of my parents' beautiful home, where they have lived for 27 years. We didn't grow up here. They moved to Tennessee in the '80s for eight years, then returned to Baton Rouge and bought this home. It's a big two-story home set in a lovely neighborhood. Their backyard is a forest setting filled with mature oak trees, backing up to the Amite River. The area features a beautiful lake with surrounding paths, and the path entrance is one house away. I love coming to this house, but what I love most is that they love it too. They didn't know about the lovely lake and the kids' playground next to it when they bought it, which was perfect for their nine young grandchildren. The home decor is a bit dated now and filled with antiques, but I love it, especially the guest bedroom I have designated as my room. It has my grandmother's old bedroom furniture, which is comforting and brings back great memories.

I walk up the stairs, passing all our framed formal wedding pictures, including my mom and dad's black and white portrait. They were very young—20 and 21. I glance at the picture of Jimmy and me walking down the aisle of St. Louis Cathedral in the French Quarter. It is one of my favorite pictures. Our smiles have never been brighter than on our special day. We look so young. It occurs to me that we are now past the age our parents were when we got married. It's unbelievable how fast life has flown by.

Dad has carried my big, heavy suitcase to my room and meets me in the hall, reminding me of tomorrow's neurologist appointment at 10:00 a.m. My three younger sisters will meet us there.

"Okay, let me unpack, and I'll be down soon," I tell him.

My father sits in his armchair and reads while Mom and I sit on the old green sofa and watch *Dancing with the Stars*. She is closer to the TV, and I'm on the other end. Soon, I am lying down with my feet next to her. She reaches over, puts my feet in her lap, and rubs them. I'm relaxed and grateful for this time together. We clapped after each dance performance as if we were right there in the audience. Everything about this show—the costumes, the music, the dancing, and the flamboyant judge—makes us happy. We laugh at his critiques.

"He's crazy," Mom announces, and we laugh harder.

"Y'all want some ice cream?" Dad asks as he stands up from his chair and walks to the kitchen.

"Yes!" we both pipe up. Ice cream for dinner! I love the way my parents think.

Soon, we are diving into big bowls of rocky road ice cream. Lately, Jimmy and I have been enjoying ice cream in little plastic gelato bowls we brought home from our favorite gelato place in Studio City. Of course, they charge $5.00 for the tiny bowl. Why do we take the disposable plastic bowls home to reuse? There is something fun and whimsical about eating gelato out of those little bright-colored bowls with tiny plastic spoons. The small gelato cup is a Los Angeles serving of ice cream, and this cereal bowl of ice cream my dad just handed me is a Louisiana serving.

I can see the five pounds creeping on me now. Every time I visit Louisiana, I go back with five additional pounds. It's just a given and worth every bite!

We are the first to arrive at the Neurology Clinic the following day. My younger sisters join us one by one: Shannan, Erin, a wine company rep, and my baby sister, Kelly, a doctor. I'm excited to see them, but I wish we were somewhere else, anywhere else. They all hug Mom and Dad, sit, and fill them in on their kids, trying to divert the attention away from why we are here. I stand up to hug them, and we whisper how this sucks.

The nurse calls out "Sherry Sweeney" from the entrance door, and we all walk single file to the door. As we follow the nurse back to the Doctor's office, I think to myself, *she must think this is overkill, six family members for a neurologist appointment*. The office is small, with only three chairs for the patient and family. The nurse brings two more chairs, and Kelly tells her she is okay with standing.

Good because there is no more room for another chair. We all look at each other nervously.

"Why are we here?" Mom asks just as the doctor comes marching in.

"The whole family is here," he cheerfully says as he shakes our hands. He sits behind his desk and starts questioning my mother.

"How old are you, Sherry?"

"Ummm…." as she looks around at each of us, and none respond. It is painful to watch.

"57," she finally blurts out, which is my age.

"What year were you born?"

"Hmmm… 1958."

"Who is the President?"

"Uh…..Clinton?"

"What floor are we on in this building?"

"I don't know."

"Do you know why you are here?"

"No."

Mom's eyes darted around, pleading for help, and we all stayed silent. It seems cruel, and I want to help her. We cringe as our beautiful mother fails each question. The knife of reality digs into my heart. I'm sure Dad and my sisters feel the same.

"Your wife has Alzheimer's," the doctor says to my father as if Mom isn't sitting in the room. The sadness creeps from my head to my heart, and I cry silently. I glance around at my sisters and see reality hit them like a ton of bricks. Dad seems stunned. Mom looks confused. It's not that we didn't know this was coming, but hearing the official Big A diagnosis slaps us in the face. Wake up! The elephant in the room over the last five years is now on top of us, suffocating us.

"You are lucky to have such a caring family. I've never seen anything like this. They are like a bunch of bees buzzing around you," the doctor tells Mom.

He tells us to set up an appointment with a neuropsychiatrist and come back to see him in six months. He reviews Mom's drugs on his computer, increases the dosages, and adds an anti-anxiety prescription.

"These medications will only slow the progression of the disease," he tells us before standing up.

24

We are dismissed. The much-dreaded doctor's appointment is finished.

We walk out of the office like deflated balloons. Was the doctor giving us a backhanded compliment? It seemed like an obnoxious stab. Has he never seen anything like this? Seriously? What the frick? I don't think we liked being compared to a bunch of bees. Yes, that's us, the honey bunches of bees buzzing around, trying to support our mother. I'm angry.

We all stop at the check-out counter while Dad sets up another appointment for six months from now. Why? What good will it do?

"Y'all want to go to lunch?" Kelly asks us as we step into the elevator. "Yes," Dad says, answering for Mom and me. Shannan bows out; she has to get to the office, and Erin has to see restaurant clients. Nobody talks about what just happened. The sadness settles in as we stand in the lobby, saying goodbye. We quickly hug Shannan and Erin, avoiding eye contact, knowing the first to cry would open the floodgates.

Dad, Mom, Kelly, and I walked across the parking lot to California Pizza Kitchen and settle into a booth. I ordered split pea soup with a salad. I need comfort food.

Mom orders the same. This time, she doesn't argue when the food comes. She eats the entire bowl but only picks at her salad. Dad finishes his pizza and Mom's salad. Kelly eats her flatbread pizza fast and leaves for work. We don't mention the doctor's appointment. The family unit has now been reduced to the three of us. Dad pays the bill, and we head to the parking garage. We drive home in silence with the Frank Sinatra channel on the Sirius Radio station playing "Send in the Clowns," followed by "That's Life." Thank you, Frank. Life sucks big time right now.

Back home, Dad goes to his chair in the living room. Mom and I head to our bedrooms for a nap. It's only 12:30 p.m., but we are both tired. It has been the longest morning. I just want to sleep and numb out the reality. As Mom opens her bedroom door, I stop and hug her.

"You okay, Mom?"

"I'm fine," she says, and I hear the sadness in her voice. I hug her closer.

"I love you," I whisper in her ear, choking back tears.

"I love you too, Peg, and I'm glad you are here," she says. She steps into her bedroom and shuts the door. She looks lost, and it breaks my heart.

26

As I walk up the stairs, I wonder if she grasps the finality of her diagnosis this morning or if she remembers any of it. I wish I didn't remember any of it. I crawl into my bed and begin to cry. I pull the covers over my head and pray all the prayers I learned in Catholic grade school—Our Father, Hail Mary, and Glory Be. I don't know what else to do.

My cell phone rings and wakes me up at 4:00 p.m. It's Jimmy. Oh, crap, I forgot to call him.

"How did it go?" he asks. I fill him in.

"I'm sorry. My day wasn't much better. It looks like the Universe made some decisions for us. I got laid off today."

"What?" I sit up, and my heart goes to my toes.

"Oh, my God! What happened?" I'm shocked but secretly grateful at the same time. Before he can tell me, I blurt out, "Did you get a package? Can you get unemployment?"

"Yes, both. I'm relieved. I've been miserable, and it will make life easier for us to move back to Louisiana."

I have been campaigning for over a year to move home to Louisiana. Jimmy didn't know I had prayed a week ago, pleading, begging God in tears to please let Jimmy get laid off. Ever since his parents died four years ago, I knew he had been unhappy working as a Branch Manager at a brokerage firm. It was a grind, with tons of corporate changes. It wasn't the job he had loved for so many years. I knew he wanted to quit, but I also knew that if he were laid off with a package, it would make it easier for us to plan a move home to Louisiana. Thank you, God, for answering my prayers!

Jimmy understands my desire to move home. Six months ago, we were lying in bed, and I told him I wanted to sell our home, return to Louisiana, and be there for my parents. In 2011, his mother died suddenly of lung cancer; eleven days later, his father died of Alzheimer's. The sudden shock of their deaths together back in New York slammed him emotionally. He wasn't prepared for the grief that followed, and I had no clue how to support him. As he slowly crawled his way out of the devastation, I started dealing with what was happening with my mom back in Louisiana.

Wow! My mind is spinning. This day is turning out to be a pivotal day that is changing the course of our future.

"Should I fly home?" I ask. The thought of him being alone right now is crushing.

"No, don't rush back. Be there for your parents. Enjoy the wedding and Easter with your family. I have a lot to do here if we are going to sell the condo and move back to Louisiana," he says. We say goodbye, and I love you.

I climb out of bed and walk down into the living room. Mom and Dad are watching the news as if it were just any other day.

"It's about time you woke up! I was starting to worry about you," Dad tells me.

"Jimmy just got laid off!" I announced.

"Oh, no!" Mom says.

"That's terrible," Dad states. I sit on the sofa and start to cry.

"It's a good thing. We can now move back to Louisiana," I tell them through tears, trying to convince them and myself.

"Come here and let me hold you," Mom says tenderly. She hugs me tight, then I lay my head in her lap and sob. She rubs my shoulders and comforts me. I cry for her. I cry for Dad, my sisters, and our family. I cry for Jimmy, and I cry for me.

"It's going to be okay, it's going to be okay, Peggy," she says repeatedly, and I try to believe her. I want to believe her. She's my wonderful, loving mother again, at least for this moment.

My mother could always make things better with her touch, smiles, laughter, singing, dancing, an ice cream cone from Baskin and Robbins, a bowl of her homemade vegetable soup, 7-Up on cracked ice, slices of watermelon or popsicles on a hot summer day, shopping for a new outfit, a visit wherever I was living, and a Hallmark card in the mail with a check to treat myself.

Her "feel better" list is unending, but nothing on the list will make her better today, tomorrow, or anytime in the distant future, and that is all I want right now. I want a magic wand that will make everything right again, erase her Alzheimer's, and make her whole and healthy again.

Can I be the loving daughter who comes home to face the hard times? Will I be able to navigate life in the A-Zone? At this moment, I just don't know.

Nanny's Shrimp-Stuffed Mirliton

Ingredients:

1 pound of peeled and deveined medium shrimp
4 large mirlitons (also known as Chayote, a green pear-shaped squash)
1/2 cup of onion, chopped
4 green onions, chopped
3 garlic cloves, minced
2 tablespoons of olive oil
1 cup of diced ham
¾ cup of Italian-style breadcrumbs, divided
1 Tbsp. Creole or Cajun seasoning
½ cup of shredded Parmesan cheese

Instructions:

Preheat the oven to 375°F
Cover mirlitons with water in a Dutch oven and bring to a boil, cook for 45-50 minutes until fork-tender.
Drain mirlitons in a colander and cool.
Cut each mirliton in half lengthwise, remove and discard seeds.
Carefully scoop out pulp with a tablespoon. Do not break the outside shell.
Chop pulp and set the shells aside.
Sauté the onions and garlic in olive oil for five minutes on medium-high.
Add shrimp and ham and cook, stirring constantly, for 3 to 5 minutes or until shrimp turn pink.
Stir in the mirliton pulp, ½ cup of breadcrumbs, and Creole seasoning, cooking for 5 minutes.
Stuff mixture evenly into mirliton shells.
Place in a lightly greased 13" x 9" baking dish.

Sprinkle the remaining ¼ cup of breadcrumbs and Parmesan cheese.
Bake at 375°F for 15 to 20 minutes.

Yield

Serves: 8

Family Notes:

This was my grandmother's recipe, and we served this for Thanksgiving or Christmas dinner as a side dish. My sister Erin has taken over this recipe and makes a casserole instead of stuffing the shells. It is delicious either way.

The mirliton is a pear-shaped green squash used in many Cajun and Creole recipes and is pronounced "mel ul tawn." It is rare to find this on a menu at Louisiana restaurants, so my family loves to order it at Harbor Seafood.

CHAPTER TWO
THE LADIES WHO LUNCH

"Where do you want to go today?" Mom would ask me on the first day of my visits to my family in Baton Rouge. We would dress up and head off to shop at the Mall of Louisiana or an upscale shopping center. Afterwards, we would have a lovely lunch at one of my favorite Baton Rouge restaurants. These were our special Mother-Daughter days.

Often, and long before Alzheimer's was on our radar, as we were ready to leave, Mom would say, "I can't find my keys," and we would spend about 10 minutes looking for them. Some days her purse was missing.

"I found them!" Dad would say.

"Where?"

"On the counter, next to your purse!"

"Do you have money?" my dad would ask her as he pulled out his money clip, handing her a bunch of bills.

"Y'all have fun today!" he would say as we headed out the door.

Mom would get behind the wheel of her "Grand Mommy Van," and we would go to Talbots, Chico's, Ann Taylor, Macy's, or Dillard's for endless shopping possibilities. I cherished these Mother-Daughter dates with her.

"Try that on. I think it will look cute on you," Mom would say as we pulled outfit after outfit off the racks. My arm would ache under the weight of the clothes until the saleswoman would rescue me and place them in a dressing room.

Sometimes Mom would find something for herself, but usually, it was all about me on those days. After about an hour of selecting clothes, we would head to the dressing room, and she would sit in the chair or bench while I tried on dresses for about thirty minutes. With each outfit, she would zip me up, give me her honest opinion, unzip me, and put the clothes back on the hanger, organizing rejections on one side of the dressing room and favorites on the other. The conversations always went something like this:

"I'm so fat. I need to go on a diet!" I'd say.

"You look great. Stop it."

"What do you think?" I asked, spinning around the too-crowded dressing room before stepping to check myself in the full-length mirror at the end of the hall.

"Peggy, take that off. The dress does nothing for you!"

"Look, Mom, this is fabulous!"

"I love it, Peg. You need to get it."

"Yes, but it's not on sale. It's full price and too expensive for me."

"I will buy it for you—it's your early birthday present, Easter, Christmas, anniversary," or she would simply say, "I haven't bought you anything for a while; I want to get this for you!"

"This shirt is cute on me."

"It looks Maw Maw," which was her word for frumpy.

"I love this dress."

"I can't get it to zip up, Peg. You need to lose a couple of pounds. Try this one. I think it will be your favorite," handing me something I would have never chosen. Bingo! My mom was always right.

"It's amazing!"

We would walk out with half of the clothes I had tried on, and she would hand me two of the sale items at the register counter.

"You can get these for yourself, and I will get the rest," she would say, pulling out her credit card. Then, as she placed her wallet back into her purse, she would hand me a wad of cash. "This is for you to use on your trip while you are here!" And off we would go to lunch, bags in hand.

My three sisters would usually join us for lunch since this was our first opportunity to get together on these trips back home. It was our special "Ladies Who Lunch" day, and I loved every minute.

Mom and I were always on the lookout for sales and bargains. Once while shopping in L.A. at the now-defunct Robinson's May department store in Beverly Hills, my friend Eugenie found a gold lame long halter dress marked down countless times to $7.50. Eugenie is 6'1", an actress, and a model who could make a grocery bag look great. She strolled out, smashing, modeling the dress for Mom and me. Other shoppers stopped in their tracks and looked at my beautiful friend. We told her she needed to get the dress, and strangers agreed. When she went to the counter to pay for the dress, it rang 50% off the $7.50, so she bought it for $3.75. Such a deal!

"If you stand here long enough, they will give it to you," Mom announced loudly for the entire women's department to hear. We laughed along with the sales associate and all the customers standing at the counter. Eugenie has worn that dress many times and says she remembers my mom's funny remarks and laughs whenever she puts it on.

During another shopping trip, when both my old New York roommate, Sherry, and my parents were visiting, Sherry joined Mom and me for our shopping trip. Since my mom's name is Sherry, too, they had a special kinship when they met in New York in the late '80s. They always giggled together over the craziest things. Having them both in Los Angeles was a treat and a blessing. Sherry picked out several cute outfits as we plundered through the sales items at Robinson's May. She was still single, living in New York in the last semester of getting her college degree, and struggling financially. This trip to Los Angeles to see her sister and me stretched her budget. Mom took the clothing out of her hand at the counter, put it on our stack, and paid for it.

My mom was a Mama Bear to everyone. Besides being fun-loving, she is the Giving Tree to the nth degree. She makes everyone feel special and loved. Years later, Sherry met her future husband, Steve, online, and when they planned their wedding in the Florida Keys, my parents were invited and joined me. Dad brought his video camera, and my parents interviewed Sherry and Steve in our hotel room, asking them how they met, their first date, where they first kissed, and what they loved most about each other.

A few years ago, my parents visited us in Los Angeles the day after Christmas and stayed through New Year's Day. Mom and I hit the mall one afternoon while Jimmy and Dad watched a football bowl game. While browsing the shoe sale at Coldwater Creek, I stumbled upon some cute cowboy boots in red with black trim and a pair of brown with tan trim.

"Try those on," Mom said, looking over my shoulder. I sat in a chair and pulled them on. I pranced around modeling them both.

She laughed when I said, "Yeehaw," side-kicking my legs in the air.

"What color should I get?" I asked her.

"I like them both," she replied.

"Let me think about it. The brown ones would be more practical. But the red ones are more me," I said as I walked into the dressing room to try on some clothes. Mom sat down in a chair.

"Your daughter needs to get the red boots," an older gentleman told Mom as he waited for his wife in the dressing room.

Mom marched into the dressing room, pulled back the curtain, and announced, "We've got this nice man's opinion. The red ones. I'll buy them for you," and grabbed the red boots and headed to the counter to pay for them.

I wear those red boots with the black trim with pride and get compliments everywhere I go. They are my happy boots! They look great on Christmas afternoon when we gather for gumbo with my family. I'm styling a Christmas sweater, blue jeans or black leggings, and my red cowboy boots. The boots make me feel sassy, and I remember that day in L.A. as if it were yesterday. I've had those boots for probably ten years now. I had them re-heeled for more than the boots cost. I can't imagine the day they fall apart, and I pitch them into the Goodwill pile. I hope that day never comes.

Since Jimmy and I moved back to Louisiana, Mom and I are now shopping with our unwelcome friend, Alzheimer's. I don't have the playbook for this new life in the A-Zone. I'm doing my best one day at a time, but it is not easy. It has been a couple of months since we moved back to Baton Rouge, and today Mom and I are walking around Macy's looking at the summer sales racks. I found a cute dress and dashed into a dressing room to try it on. She sits on a chair outside the dressing room, holding a $100 bag of expensive department store makeup on her lap. She couldn't find her makeup this morning, so my father told me to take her shopping. The saleswoman matched her skin for the foundation, then she picked out a pink lipstick and powder, spending enough to get the gift with purchase.

The dress is way too tight! Damn! I've had too much Louisiana food these past few months. I quickly changed. As I walked out of the dressing room, I noticed Mom is gone. Oh no!

"Mom?" I call out repeatedly, dashing through the aisles of Women's Wear, then continuing into the lingerie department, looking right and left.

"Mom?"

I am now in full-blown panic! WTF!

My phone rang. It's my sister, Erin. "Where are y'all? I'm here in Macy's."

"I lost Mom."

"Oh, my God!" she replied.

We stay on the phone with each other as she checks the shoe department, and I head to the jewelry department, where I find my mother talking to a sales associate. She looks confused and flustered.

"Where did you go? You left me," she snaps at me.

"I'm sorry, Mom. I came out of the dressing room, and you were gone."

I realize mid-sentence that this is hopeless. There is no explanation. She's lost in the Alzheimer's maze. My mom, who could navigate any department store with her four little girls trailing behind her, is reduced to being a scared little child being led around by her clueless daughter. I feel like a total loser. I'm lost in the Alzheimer's maze too!

Erin walks up, and we look at each other, relieved. I'm defeated. I lost my mom. What the hell was I thinking? Thank God she didn't walk out of the store. I'm a nervous wreck. I can't wait to get out of here.

"Let's go have lunch at Cheesecake Bistro," Erin suggests. She knows I'm upset, and she takes charge. We sat in a big booth. I hold back tears while Erin chats with Mom in her perky way for most of the lunch. I'm grateful she is here with us. I stab at my shrimp salad, stuffing my face, barely tasting it. I butter a French roll, eat it, and butter another. I'm eating my feelings.

We drove back home in silence, listening to the '50s station on Sirius Radio. I'm her designated driver these days, navigating her van. Mom hasn't driven since she was officially diagnosed with Alzheimer's.

"Did y'all have a good time?" Dad asks as we walk into the house. Mom doesn't say anything. She walks to their bedroom and closes the door. I tell my father about losing Mom. He rolls his eyes, shakes his head, and says, "I'm sorry."

I head upstairs, crawl into our bed, my refuge, and cry. My tears seem endless these days. I come downstairs a few hours later, and Mom sits in the living room with Dad. She looks pissed off.

"Your mom can't find the makeup she bought today. Do you have it?" he asks.

We look in the car, their bedroom, bathrooms, closets, and the kitchen. I even searched our bedroom, thinking maybe I had it. Dad is frustrated, and I'm on the verge of screaming. We finally found the bag in their laundry cabinet, shoved behind some dirty clothes.

"How did it get there? I didn't put it there," Mom said.

"I don't know, Mom," I say, turning and heading to the kitchen to cook dinner. I feel like I'm going mad. Dad comes into the kitchen and pours himself a glass of wine. We look at each other and just shake our heads.

"I'm sorry," he says again. My father is constantly apologizing for Mom's behavior to me.

"Yeah, me too, Dad," and we hugged. It seems like it's us against my mom in the A-Zone. We are struggling in the A-Zone, and I can't imagine the bleak future.

Since I moved back home, we have been shopping at least once a week at the mall. My mother is no longer buying me clothes, so I'm spending money on unnecessary items just to get her out of the house because she is restless and says she wants to "go somewhere." Dad gives her cash now when we leave. He gives me money for our lunch, and off we go for a few hours. At the store, she tells me, "I have no money!" I opened her wallet to show her the money. She hands the woman at the cash register three $20 bills for a twelve-dollar purchase. The woman looks at me, and I step back behind Mom, roll my eyes, and shake my head. She gives two $20 bills back to Mom and then hands her the change. Mom is confused and doesn't know what to do with all the money. I realize she can no longer count. Another check in the A-Zone box.

She hardly ever wears the new clothes she buys. I pull them out, suggesting she wear them, and she tells me she doesn't like them.

One day, we passed a Goodwill Store, and I pulled in impulsively.

"What are we doing here?" she sneers.

"Let's go look around, Mom."

"Really?"

"Sure. It will be fun. Who knows what we will find?" I say in my most convincing voice.

Genius! We spent forty-five minutes wandering around and found a few nice things from some of our favorite stores, Chico's and Ann Taylor. She likes it. I have never understood the draw of resale shops, even though I have thrift-obsessed friends. Now, I search for every Goodwill in Baton Rouge and even discover another local thrift store called The Purple Cow. We hit them all, becoming thrift store shoppers just like that. Instead of spending $60-$100 per shopping visit at the mall, we pay $5 to $10, and we love it! Thrift shopping has become our new thing.

We find cute shirts, jackets, dresses, and some lovely pants. Some of the items Mom picks out are strange, like a wicker suitcase she has never used. It just sits on the top shelf of our laundry closet.

Mom continues to lose her makeup, and it is a daily source of anxiety. We stop buying high-end cosmetics and head to the Dollar Tree. We fill a green plastic basket with lipsticks, powder, eyeshadow, eyebrow pencils, brushes, and combs. She loses it all, and we head back to Dollar Tree a week later.

The latest missing item is a pair of scissors. We know they are in the house somewhere, but nobody can find them. Dollar Tree has scissors for a buck, so now Dad takes her there at least twice a month to buy scissors.

I finally snatched one of the pairs and put them in the kitchen utensil drawer instead of the desk drawer, a simple solution that took me months to figure out.

Mom and Dad soon discover the candy aisle at the dollar store and come back with movie candy-sized boxes of hot tamales, M&M's, Junior Mints, Starburst, and Raisinets.

"It's our movie candy," they say, and add it to Mom's overflowing black purse when they go to the movie theatre. They stash the candy in the table linen drawer, "hiding" it from Jimmy and me. They know Jimmy loves Junior Mints and Raisinets.

One night, the candy calls to me after a particularly tough day with Mom. She is pissed off at Dad and hiding in her room with the door locked. She forgets he has a key over the door frame and can open it anytime.

I knock on her door. "Mom, you want to come out and watch *The Voice* with me?" I wait and knock again. She opens the door, standing like a little child.

"Sure," she says.

We find our spots on the old green sofa. Mom sits on the end closest to the TV. I lay with my head on the other end, my feet in her lap. It's my go-to spot. We soon get caught up in the show, clapping and laughing. Finally, I give in to the candy urge, jump up, and go to the secret stash drawer. Yes, there it is, my favorite, Peanut M&M's under the rarely used placemats and cloth napkins. I grab the box,

46

open the tightly sealed plastic with my hidden scissors, and head to the den. I hand her fistfuls of candy, and while we cheer for our favorite singers, we get our sugar fix.

From the mall to Goodwill, Purple Cow, and Dollar Tree, our shopping outings have become shorter. The ladies who lunch rarely go out to lunch anymore. Soon, my mother, who was pacing the house, anxious to "go somewhere," is only happy going out for about an hour. We ride around the area, and sometimes she doesn't even want to get out of the car at Dollar Tree. I'm scared to leave her in the car alone; afraid she will wander off.

"Do you want to go out to lunch?" I continue to ask.

"No, we can eat at home. I want to go check on Dad."

The shopping trips slipped away just like my mom slipped away, I think, as I turned the box of candy upside down. The last peanut M&M's rolls out, and I hand it to her. She smiles at me and says, "Thank you, Peg."

As hard as this is, I realize I'm doing the right thing. I missed so many good times when she was fully present, but tonight, I am here, fully present for our Life in the A-Zone—savoring it like that last peanut M&M's.

CHAPTER THREE
MEATBALL MADNESS

"Your mom wants to make her meatballs and spaghetti for you and Jimmy!" Dad announces as he pulls out our Nanny Cookbook, looking for the recipe.

My sisters, Shannan and Kelly, created our family cookbook many years ago. It was a massive project with pictures and recipes from our grandmothers, moms, aunts, mothers-in-law, cousins, sisters, nieces, and friends. The pink cover features a beautiful black and white picture of our beautiful grandmother, "Nanny," likely taken in her early 20s. We all received these special cookbooks for Christmas that year and have given them to our friends over the years. We cherish the cookbook as our go-to for any old family recipes.

Dad flips through the cookbook, finds the recipe, writes down a grocery list of items for the meatballs and sauce, and then gets ready to head to the grocery store as soon as Mom can find her purse, which could take anywhere from five to thirty minutes.

"I can help cook when I get back later today," I say, dashing out the door.

At three o'clock, I begin pulling out the recipe items: packs of Italian sausage, ground meat, onions, celery, bell peppers, green onions, garlic, olive oil, salt, pepper, Italian seasonings, breadcrumbs, eggs, and jars of tomato sauce. I turn to the meatball recipe in the Nanny cookbook and notice it is not Mom's recipe, but someone else's. Damn! I must have missed out, as I never remember Mom making these meatballs. I've never made meatballs, but I'm up for the task.

Mom joins me in the kitchen. I set up chopping boards on the counter. Dad comes in, grabs a knife, a board, and onions, and sits at the table to chop the onions. Mom stands at the counter, and I give her the celery. I start uncasing the sausage and look over to see her chopping large slices of celery.

"Mom, you need to chop the celery smaller," I say without thinking.

"What's wrong with these slices?"

"Too big for meatballs. You need to chop it finely."

She throws her hands up in the air dramatically and says, "You do it!"

"Mom!"

"You take over my car, my house, my kitchen, and now you are telling me how to cook!" she says, storming to her bedroom and slamming the door.

"What happened?" Dad asked. He wasn't paying attention to the interaction before the outburst. He is hard of hearing, and his hearing aids are clearly NOT working today, a source of constant frustration. I fill him in on the testy situation and stand there, totally frustrated. I walk to the bedroom door, find the door locked, and knock.

"I'm sorry, Mom. Please come back. I didn't mean to hurt your feelings. Tonight was supposed to be a fun mother-daughter bonding dinner. I need your help," I beg through the locked door.

I get no response! Dad comes down the hall and stands behind me. He sees that I'm about to start to cry.

"Sherry, please come to the kitchen and help Peggy make your meatballs," he begs.

"Yeah, Mom, I've never made meatballs! I have no idea what I'm doing," I say sweetly with tears in my voice.

Nada! Total Silence. WTF! Jimmy walks in the back door and hears the commotion in the hall.

"What's going on?"

I tell him the problem, and he shakes his head and heads upstairs.

"Cuckoo for Coco Puffs!" he says under his breath. He is not getting in the middle of the meatball madness.

I guess I'm making meatballs on my own. They bought about five pounds of sausage and ground meat, and with all the chopped seasoning, it now fills a huge aluminum bowl. So now I'm crying and up to my elbows, mixing the slimy meatball mixture with my hands. I hate the consistency, which is probably why I've never made meatballs!

I wish we were back in L.A. having a take-out meatball dinner! Back in Los Angeles, Jimmy and I would purchase incredible meatballs and sauce from a cute Italian Deli called Bay Cities, which also offered homemade pasta and the best Italian bread ever. It would be impossible to find parking in their lot. You had to pull a number at the counter and wait forever before being served, but their meatballs and homemade pasta reminded Jimmy of his favorite New York Italian restaurants.

I can't catch my tears or wipe my runny nose, so I cock my head down while lifting my shoulder, wiping both with my shirt. Lovely!

Dad comes over and stands at the counter, watching me.

"Can you help me roll them, Dad?" I ask. He looks at the meatballs I have rolled so far.

"You're making them too big," he advises, and I give him a look.

Seriously? Don't start with me, I think to myself. We stand together silently, rolling countless meatballs and placing them on large cookie sheets filled with parchment paper.

While Dad places the trays in the oven to bake, I go to the bedroom door and knock again. I beg Mom one more time to please join me. No response. Frick it! This situation sucks big time. I head back to the kitchen to start the sauce. Soon, the house smells fantastic.

I boil the pasta, toss a green salad, and prepare garlic bread.

Realizing we will have meatballs for days and Mom probably won't join us for dinner, I have a great idea! Sweeney sisters to the rescue. I text them on the "Sisters" text thread.

Dinner? Mom wanted to make her meatballs. Now pissed at me and locked in her bedroom.

Oh no! Rob's working late, but I'm down for some meatballs! What time? Shannan texts.

Scott, Peyton, and I will come for meatballs. I'll bring some wine and some champagne to make Mom a mimosa! Erin texts.

I can't make it tonight. Girls have ballet. Duncan has homework but save me some meatballs. When did Mom start making meatballs? Kelly texts.

7:00 p.m. is good. I don't remember Mom ever making meatballs. I text back.

Mom made spaghetti and meat sauce, never meatballs! Shannan texts.

The Big A lightbulb goes off. OMG! Mom meant to say she wanted to make meat sauce and spaghetti, not meatballs and spaghetti. Holy crap! I was clueless, and Dad was too!

Shannan, Erin, my brother-in-law Scott, and my niece Peyton arrive, and they walk through the kitchen straight to the bedroom door and knock.

"Mom, we're here for dinner," Shannan yells through the door as she knocks three times.

"Come out, Mom. I'm making you a mimosa," Erin pleads, knocking three more times.

Within seconds, my mother comes bouncing out with a smile, happy to see them and her precious granddaughter, Peyton. Dad has set the kitchen table, which has only six chairs, and they all sit down—Mom, Dad, Shannan, Erin, Scott, and Peyton. I serve them steaming plates with my beautiful meatballs and sauce on the spaghetti. They pass the salad. Jimmy brings them the breadbasket. There's no room for us at the table, so Jimmy and I sit at the counter on barstools, the "kiddie counter" where the grandkids usually sit!

"These are delicious!"

"Yummy!"

"So good, Peg."

"Thanks for inviting us over!" They all comment as they eat my delicious spaghetti and meatballs.

Jimmy and I sit and eat in silence. I stuff my face even though I'm so upset that I have lost my appetite. I'm eating these frickin meatballs!

They are laughing, telling stories, drinking wine, and lapping up my luscious spaghetti and meatballs! I glanced at Mom sipping her mimosa. I haven't seen her this animated in weeks. She hasn't looked at me once and is giving me the cold shoulder. Does she even remember why she is mad at me?

"Do we have dessert?" Erin asks.

"No dessert!" Jimmy barks annoyingly.

They finish eating and move into the living room with their drinks. Jimmy and I scoop the leftover meatballs into plastic containers, since everyone wants to take home leftovers. We set aside a container for Kelly, too. There are now only eight meatballs left for us. We clear the table and start cleaning the messy kitchen. I hear them laughing and having a great time. Tears roll down my face as I load the dishwasher. I feel left out and ignored.

"Well, at least you know how to make meatballs with sauce now!" Jimmy says as he stands washing the big pot and makes me laugh with the way he says "sauce" with his New York accent.

"Red gravy," I replied through my tears, and we laughed at a running joke between us. When we lived in New Orleans in the '90s, we always heard the locals call spaghetti sauce "red gravy."

"That is just wrong. You can't call spaghetti sauce red gravy," Jimmy would say, annoyed.

Soon, they leave carrying their plastic containers of meatballs. Mom turns and walks away in silence to her bedroom, and I hear the door shut.

We are dismissed. I don't get a goodnight hug from Mom, nor a thank you for dinner.

"Well, that was a shit show," Jimmy says as he takes the garbage out before settling on our carport to smoke a cigar. The carport cigar lounge has become his escape from the A-Zone, his little bit of sanity!

"Thanks, Peg! Good job with dinner. Everyone enjoyed dinner," Dad says, before settling into his chair in the living room to lose himself in a good book. Reading is his escape from the A-Zone.

Despite the meatball madness, they were fricken amazing, and the seasoning was chopped just right. And, I haven't made meatballs since!

Mom's Spaghetti and Meat Sauce

Ingredients:

1 pound of lean ground beef
2 tbsp. Olive oil
1 medium yellow onion, chopped
4 cloves of minced garlic
1 medium bell pepper, chopped
1 24 oz. jar of Tomato Basil Spaghetti Sauce
1 14.5 oz. can of diced tomatoes with garlic and onion
One tsp. Italian seasoning
Salt, Black Pepper, and crushed red pepper flakes to taste
One-pound bag of spaghetti

Instructions:

In a large pot, sauté onions and bell pepper in olive oil until softened.
Add garlic and ground beef and cook until the meat is brown.
Add a 24-ounce jar of spaghetti sauce and a 16-ounce can of chopped tomatoes.
Add to taste: Italian seasoning, salt, black pepper, and red pepper flakes.
Cook for 15 minutes on medium, then simmer for 30 minutes.
Cook pasta according to the package.
Save 1/2 cup of pasta water before draining and add the water to the sauce.

Serve

Ladle meat sauce over pasta with grated parmesan cheese.
Serve with buttered green peas, green salad, and garlic bread.

Yield

Serves Six. (The recipe can be doubled or tripled for large parties)

Family Notes:

The meat sauce is better the second day. We always have peas with our spaghetti—it's a Sweeney thing. My husband, Jimmy, thinks it's the weirdest combination, but we love it! My Italian friends roll their eyes when we use Spaghetti Sauce from a jar, but it's the easier, softer way. If you want to make your own red sauce, go for it! With four daughters all running around to dance class, play rehearsals, and various clubs, Mom was the queen of whipping up a fast supper within an hour! We also grew up on frozen pot pies and TV dinners when my parents went out to dinner at Fairwood Country Club on weekends. We considered it a treat! I especially loved the meatloaf dinner with mashed potatoes and spiced apples.

CHAPTER FOUR
PINK CLOUD MOMENTS

"Let the sunshine in!" I announce one morning as I find Mom and Dad sitting in the living room, drinking coffee with all the blinds closed. Their living room has three walls of windows that look out to a beautiful forest setting backyard, including a deck and a fountain. It's my favorite room in the house, filled with sunlight when the blinds are open, but it feels gloomy and suffocating when they are closed. It is not a good atmosphere for dealing with my mom's Alzheimer's and my lingering depression. I walk around the room, turning the rods to open the blinds—three windows for each wall, with nine sets of blinds. Opening the blinds is how I start my morning routine for our life in the A-Zone.

I finally broke down and made an appointment today to see Dr. April, my mom's general practitioner. Mom loves

Dr. April, and I am impressed with her sweet bedside manner. She referred us to the neurologist and has been on this journey with our family since we first noticed Mom's memory loss. She is also a family friend, going back to when she babysat my sister's kids while she was in college.

Waiting in the small office, I realize I am ready to surrender. I need help. I can't deal with this on my own. I'm anxious, can't sleep at night, and feel depressed.

"Hi, Peggy. I was surprised to see your name on the list today. How are you?" Dr. April says to me.

"I'm a mess," and I burst into tears. She hands me some tissues and sits across from me.

"Of course you are. You are living with Alzheimer's. It's tough."

I leave with a hug and prescriptions for anxiety, sleeplessness, and depression. I feel weak, broken, and defeated. I'm grateful for Dr. April's compassion and understanding. It was a relief to have her inform me that falling apart is normal for caregivers.

I stop at the drugstore counter at our local grocery store and drop off the prescriptions. I decided to have tomato soup for lunch. Campbell's Tomato Soup is the ultimate comfort food. I fill a plastic handbasket with the soup, a quart of milk, sliced American cheese, and saltine crackers.

As the pharmacist hands over my bag of pills, she smiles at me and tells me to have a good day. She is the same pharmacist who fills my mom's meds. I wonder if she sees this regularly, family caregivers who eventually break down and come in for their own meds. I am now officially a medicated caregiver. I've joined the club. I surrender. Life in the A-Zone is kicking my ass and sucking my soul. I sometimes wonder if I will ever feel like myself again. My mom's disease is hammering me.

Arriving home, I discover Mom is sleeping in her bed, and Dad is upstairs in his office. Now 81, my dad is still working. He has his own recruiting company and places people worldwide in the industrial sales industry. He loves helping people find jobs, especially those who have been laid off. My dad can relate to the dismay of a layoff. After 37 years, he was given a package and showed the door. He turned around, opened his own company, and never looked back. With my mom's Alzheimer's, it has become harder and harder for him to work. He goes to his office to call clients and send emails, but Mom has no sense of time and thinks he has been upstairs all day, even if it has only been fifteen minutes.

"What are you doing up there? Nobody cares about me," she hollers from the bottom of the stairs.

"I'm working, Sherry. I will be down soon. Please just give me a few more minutes," he hollers back.

"You've been up there for hours," she replies defiantly.

He finishes his work, hurries downstairs to fix her lunch, takes her for a ride to Dairy Queen for a Blizzard shake, watches TV, or plays old family movies, anything to pass the time. He is grateful when she takes naps so he can escape to his tiny office at the top of the stairs.

Today, I find it very sad that Mom is already taking a nap at 11:00 a.m. My mom never napped before Alzheimer's. I open the bedroom door, and she is staring at the wall.

"Mom, are you okay? Are you hungry? I'm going to make some tomato soup," I say sweetly as I walk over to her side of the bed.

"Hi. That sounds good," Mom says listlessly. I sit on her bed, lean down, and kiss her. I touch her hair tenderly. She needs color, but her hairdresser appointments are rare these days. She has no patience to wait while the color processes in her hair and gives her hairdresser a hard time, so it's just not worth it. I touch up her roots with the magic hair powder if we have somewhere nice to go.

I helped her get out of bed. She is dressed but has a short robe over her clothes. She is always cold these days.

"Where's Dad?" she asks.

"Upstairs working," I reply.

"He's always working," she says sadly.

She sits at the kitchen table while I make canned tomato soup with milk, just like she made it for me as a child. It is our favorite. She used to unwrap sliced American cheese and place it on the hot soup to melt, so I do that now. Once it melts, I swirl it around with a spoon and add lots of black pepper, which she loves. I brought her soup, saltine crackers, and an iced tea. I sit and join her with my bowl of soup. This simple meal brings me comfort, and I hope it brings her some, too.

I glance out the kitchen window and see a bright pink blanket of azaleas on the bushes in the backyard. Blooming azaleas are a sign that spring has sprung in Baton Rouge. This burst of pink is just what we need today!

"Look, Mom, the azaleas are in bloom!" I said, surprising myself with the excitement in my voice. The beautiful hot pink azaleas are our lifeline today—a spark in our dull day, a distraction from the gloom surrounding us like an oppressive gray blanket.

"They are beautiful!" she says and smiles. Her smiles are rare these days.

"After lunch, let's go outside and take pictures by the azaleas."

I clear the dishes from the kitchen table and walk her back to her bedroom to remove her robe.

"Let's find something pink for you to wear in the pictures," I say, opening her closet door. I found a bright pink jacket with black trim. It is a perfect pink to match the azaleas.

"This is perfect, Mom. You will match the flowers."

"I have to put this on? Really?" she says and laughs at me as I make her change into the pretty pink jacket.

"Let's put some make-up on."

She follows me into her bathroom and sits at her vanity. I started primping her with powder, blush, eye shadow, mascara, and pink lipstick. I brush her hair and fix the roots with the brown magic powder.

"What are y'all doing?" Dad asks as he comes down the stairs and hears us in the bathroom.

"We are going to take pictures outside by the azaleas! I'm Mom's make-up artist and hairdresser. I left some tomato soup on the stove for you for lunch."

"Thanks. Sounds great."

I pose Mom in front of the azaleas and take pictures with my iPhone. She smiles, and we laugh together. I snapped a few selfies with both of us. The images of Mom are beautiful. She looks healthy, vibrant, and alive. Her eyes are sparkling. In this precious moment of grace, it's like old times. However, I look pale and disheveled, with mascara from crying at the doctor's office under my eyes. I look lifeless. I should have done my makeup and hair over again. My gray roots are showing. I need that magic hair powder.

I texted the pictures of Mom to my sisters.

Gorgeous!

So cute!

Save that picture! They texted back.

We sat in the living room on the big green sofa, viewing the images on my phone.

"Look, Mom! You are gorgeous!" She smiles, and I can tell she likes her photos.

"My mama loved pink!" she says.

"I know. It was Nanny's favorite color," I say, just as a loud noise from the bookshelf startles us, and we both look up.

"What was that?" I say as I walk over to the bookshelf.

"I don't know," she says.

"A picture frame fell over. That's weird," I say, lifting a wooden picture frame that had fallen face forward onto the shelf. It's a photo of my grandmother, Nanny, in a pink shirt holding my newborn niece, Peyton, years ago. I walk over and show it to Mom.

"She's here. My Mom's here!" Mom says, and I know it is true.

***

To understand my mother, you have to know the woman who came before her. Nanny, as we called our grandmother, was full of life and a shining soul. My mother inherited her love of life, family, and food, which she passed on to us. We were lucky to have such a young and loving grandmother.

Belle Vidrine was a spunky redhead, a Cajun from Ville Platte, Louisiana, and the third youngest of ten children. When she was ten years old, her mother passed away from blood poisoning from a splinter in her foot, leaving behind a newborn baby boy, Louis, and a five-year-old daughter, Euna Mae, for Nanny to mother as the rest of the kids were out working in the fields or married and gone. She quickly took charge of her siblings and the household. At fifteen, her sharecropper father sent her to live in New Orleans with her cousins. He thought it would be a better life for her. Within months, she was married and pregnant with my mother. Poppy, our grandfather, was Irish and grew up in New Orleans. He died at 49 of lung cancer when I was seven, and I don't have many memories of him.

Growing up, our trips to New Orleans from Baton Rouge to visit Nanny were a treat, especially in the summer when I would spend a week with her. Sometimes I would go alone or with my sisters. My cousin, Siobhan, who lived in New Orleans, would always stay with us, along with Tammy, a young girl my age whom Nanny babysat and who we loved like a sister.

Nanny would plan endless activities for us. Our days were filled with walks down St. Charles Avenue to the Audubon Zoo, watching the seals being fed, or riding the streetcar to Canal Street to shop and have lunch at Maison Blanche. We played with dolls, Barbies, marbles, and jacks on the front porch. Sometimes, we would rendezvous with our Vidrine cousins–Jeanne, Mark, Barbara, and Suzanne, and go crabbing in the local canals.

We leaned over the water with chicken necks tied to big crab nets, hoping to catch dinner. My sister Shannan remembers Nanny walking out on the large pipes that crossed the canal to tie crab nets, hoping for a better catch. She was fearless!

We picnicked with bologna or ham sandwiches on white bread with mayo, Creole mustard, potato chips, or Cheetos and Little Debbie cakes for dessert. We returned home with a few small crabs, which we played with on the back driveway. Sweaty and exhausted, Nanny would set up a small plastic pool and a slip-and-slide in the backyard for us to cool off while she stood at the stove in her tiny kitchen, fixing our favorite meals. She was an excellent cook, and everything she made—gumbo, chicken fricassee, shrimp creole, red beans and rice, white beans, okra, and more—was all delicious.

"Do you want a little pusher?" Nanny would ask us, pulling out sliced white bread with tubbed margarine to sop up all the leftover gravy on our plates.

For breakfast, she would fry eggs, make a big pot of buttered grits, and serve hot biscuits with her homemade fig jam from the fig tree in the backyard. A hot buttered biscuit with fig jam and a glass of milk is still one of my all-time favorite breakfasts, and my mouth waters just thinking about it!

Some mornings, we piled into her Volkswagen Beetle and drove to McKenzie's Bakery for hot donuts with small cartons of milk to consume in the car. We would bring home Doberge cake squares in different flavors for dessert that night - coconut, chocolate, and strawberry. Some nights after dinner, we would cram into the Beetle with the sunroof open, and she would take us to the local snowball stand for bright pink nectar snowballs, a New Orleans specialty, laced with condensed milk on top.

Our favorite treat was driving out to Lake Pontchartrain, where watermelon was sold by the slice next to the Mardi Gras Fountain. The water jets lit up in shifting colors every few seconds. It felt magical. We raced around the giant fountain, then settled on the steps that led straight into the lake, eating our watermelon sprinkled with salt, the wind spraying our faces, and the waves crashing at our feet.

One night, lightning flashed across the sky and thunder rumbled in the distance, but we were having too much fun to leave. Then, in true Louisiana fashion, the heavens opened up with torrential sideways rain.

Back home, Nanny would draw a hot bath with Mr. Bubbles. Two at a time, we'd climb in, then slip into our cute summer pajamas. She always smoothed Cherry Jergens lotion onto our arms and legs, then dusted us with baby powder, the sweet scent clinging to us as we curled up fresh and clean, ready for the music to begin.

Nanny loved music. She played Dean Martin and Frank Sinatra albums on the big stereo console in her living room. She taught us how to jitterbug to "In the Mood." She told us how she met Dean Martin at the Maison Blanche store when he was in town, and he kissed her hand. She swore she didn't wash it for a week!

She only had a small one-bedroom apartment. When we visited, she'd set up our sleeping bags in the living room for some of us, while two would curl up on the sofa – heads at opposite ends, legs tangled in the middle. It felt like a slumber party, and we giggled late into the night.

71

Nanny would take the Greyhound Bus to visit us in Baton Rouge several times a year. Mom would let her take over the kitchen, and Dad couldn't get enough of her great dinners. Late at night, she would sneak upstairs with little Dixie cups of 7-Up and Sara Lee brownies on a tray. It was our little secret.

Nanny loved pink, and pink became the color of the world for her granddaughters, nieces, and Tammy. She kept a hot pink suitcase filled with dolls and doll clothes under her bed for us to play with. At Easter, she bought us baby chicks dyed in pastel colors, and we fought over who would claim the pink one. We spent hours decorating Easter eggs— mostly pink. She always bought us matching pink pajamas. She made us pink Shirley Temples with cherries, and we sat sipping them like princesses on the porch for happy hour with paper plates of cubed cheese and grapes while she drank her whiskey sour with a maraschino cherry. Her bedspread was a pale pink chenille, and her bathroom had a pink shower curtain and rug. With Nanny, life was always wrapped in pink!

Thirty-three years later, the pink faded. Jimmy and I were at a wedding in Florida when my mother called to tell me Nanny was dying and in hospice care in New Orleans. We quickly changed our tickets to fly back to Louisiana instead of the other L.A.—Los Angeles. Arriving in New Orleans the next day, we rented a car and drove straight to the hospital. My mother had just left to drive home to Baton Rouge. She wanted to go home to shower and get clean clothes. Jimmy stayed with me for an hour, then left to meet an old friend. I was now alone with Nanny. On morphine, she drifted in and out, her breaths turning ragged and strange.

"Why is she making that awful sound?" I asked the nurse.

"That's the death rattle," he said gently. "All her organs are shutting down. It won't be long." He adjusted her IV with another dose of morphine. When he left, I climbed into bed beside her and wrapped my arm around her.

"I love you, Nanny. It's okay to go." I whispered to her.

Aunt Mae, Uncle Willie, and Uncle Louis arrived, and I quickly climbed out of bed. They were shocked to see how their beloved sister looked. She opened her eyes and acknowledged them but kept drifting off. A Catholic priest came into the room to offer her communion, but once he saw her condition, he quietly asked if he should give her the last rites.

"Yes, please," I said—then instantly regretted not waiting for my mother. *Was this the moment? Was she dying now? Oh no! Should I call my mom?* We circled the bed, praying softly, tears slipping down our faces.

After her siblings left, she opened her eyes and stared toward the end of the bed. It seemed as if someone was standing there.

"Nanny, what are you looking at?" I asked softly.

"Nothing really," she whispered, though her eyes never wavered.

I felt certain her mother, father, and Poppy were all there waiting to take her home to heaven. It was eerie, yet strangely comforting. A few hours later, my mother arrived to spend the night with her. I kissed Nanny goodbye before Jimmy, and I drove back to Baton Rouge.

"Look at the sky, Peggy. The heavens are opening up to take your grandmother home," Jimmy said as we drove across Lake Pontchartrain.

I looked up, and the sky was brilliant pink.

"Pink. Nanny's favorite color," I whispered, tears streaming down my face.

Two hours later, Mom called to say Nanny had passed. Dad, Jimmy, and I sat up, waiting for her to come home.

"She was waiting for you, Peggy. You were her first granddaughter, and I think she wanted to see you before she passed," Mom said as she walked through the back door. We sat together on the green sofa, hugging and crying throughout the night. I told her about the pink sky and what Jimmy had said.

From that day on, whenever we see a pink sky, we exclaim, "A Nanny pink sky!" My mother always says, "My mom is here!" We then stand in the glow of the pink sky in silence, knowing we are being taken care of and watched over by our Nanny. Over the years, we have texted pictures of pink skies everywhere. The pink sky is our guidepost, and we know Nanny is watching over us. She is our guardian angel who makes everything okay.

So here I am sitting with Mom today on the old green sofa. She is wearing her bright pink jacket and holding the picture of Nanny dressed in a pink shirt, which had just slipped face down on the bookshelf. We scroll through the photos on my phone—Mom smiling in front of the pink azaleas—I realize it is a true pink cloud moment. We are blessed.

At this moment, there is no Alzheimer's, no depression, no sadness, just pure pink joy. And we are okay because we know Nanny is here.

Pink cloud moments come in many forms, if you look for them. In fact, the more you look for them, the more they appear. Today's pink cloud moment arrived in our own backyard—a blanket of brilliant hot pink azaleas. This grace didn't cost anything, and it required no effort. Yet the joy, the sweetness, and the beautiful photograph of my mother among those hot pink blooms will stay with me for the rest of my life. And for that, I am deeply grateful.

Nanny's Fig Preserves

Ingredients:

5 lbs. fresh figs, cleaned and cut in half (do not cut smaller)
Large bowl with water to soak figs
4 Tbsp. baking soda
2-½ cups of sugar
5 lemons sliced
12 Ball Jars with lids

Instructions:

Wash figs in a colander.
Soak figs in water with baking soda.
Cut stems off figs after soaking for one and ½ hours.
Put figs, sugar, and 2 cups of water in a large pot.
Cook for one and ½ hours on medium, stirring often to ensure sugar doesn't stick to the bottom of the pot.
When it begins to boil, reduce the heat to low and continue to cook until the figs are soft but not falling apart.
Add lemon slices in the last 15 minutes.

Prepare the Jars:

Scald the jars and tops in boiling water for 15 minutes.
Remove and place upside down on a towel to drain and cool.
Spoon figs and sauce with lemon slices into the jars, ensuring the lids are closed (they should make a popping noise).
Once the jars are cool, refrigerate or store them in a cool, dark pantry for up to eight months.
Once opened, they will last up to 3-4 weeks

To Serve

Spread on hot buttered biscuits or toast.

Dad's Easy Drop Biscuits

Ingredients

2-¼ cups of Original Bisquick Mix
⅔ cups of cold milk

Instructions:

Heat oven to 400°F
In a medium bowl, stir Bisquick and milk until soft dough forms.
Drop by spoonful onto an ungreased cookie sheet (They will be lumpy and don't have to look pretty)
Bake for 12 minutes or until golden brown

To Serve

Enjoy with butter and Nanny's Fig Jam.

Yield

Approximately 12-16 biscuits; serves 6-8.

Family Note:

My cousins who lived in Pennsylvania and would visit us in the summer raved about my dad's famous biscuits! They are simple but delicious.

CHAPTER FIVE
LESSONS OF THE LAKE

He stands in stillness, alone in the early-morning mist, balanced on a hidden log in the murky lake—so still it looks as if he's standing on water. I imagine him walking across to his particular spot as King of the Lake. He has been here every day for over a week, or at least every time I walk. He stands with pride and doesn't move. I stop on the footbridge that crosses the dam and watch my friend, a beautiful White Heron. He watches me back.

"Give me your strength and grace," I whisper.

It rained last night, and water rushes under the bridge and down the concrete slope of the dam into the swampy, dark Amite River below. It sounds like a waterfall—music to my ears in the silence of the morning. There are homes around the lake, but today it is quiet—no leaf blowers, no voices, no other walkers. I'm the only one on the path at the

79

south end of the Lake at White Oak, and I am grateful for this time alone.

Sunlight scatters across the surface, a million diamonds bobbing in the light. *Be still, my soul,* I whisper. I take a deep breath and pray, "God, let me carry this beauty and serenity through the rest of my day, my week, my month, my life." I turn and walk off the bridge, putting one foot in front of the other. *Stay in the moment,* I tell myself, placing my hand over my heart. This simple gesture grounds me. In this moment, I am Okay.

Later that evening, I Google the spiritual meaning of the White Heron. It speaks to wild, unspoiled beauty, purity, and patience. I take it as a sign and claim my White Heron as my spirit animal.

These days, I look for signs everywhere—crumbs of life to show me the way.

Like the White Heron, I long to feel that wildness and unspoiled beauty in my heart as I struggle with our new normal—life in Baton Rouge with my mom's Alzheimer's—our life in the A-Zone.

We are in the trenches, my dad and me. Jimmy stands in the inner circle, and my sisters stand just outside, doing what they can. It's interesting how each of us reacts differently. Denial chips away at different speeds. Dad and I are still trying to reason with her, to help her. It isn't working. Throwing our hands up and surrendering is a tricky step. We can't bring ourselves to do that yet. I WILL NOT go down with the Alzheimer's ship.

On my early-morning walks, I feel one with nature, connected to the earth. I feel peace, and when I turn into our driveway, my mantra is, "I can do this. It will be a good day." On the bad days, I walk in the afternoon with tears on my cheeks, cursing my mom's insidious disease. I pray for patience. Purity of thought feels impossible.

Sorry, White Heron—that is a lofty goal, and it's out of my reach right now.

***

Eight months ago, the waters rose—two days after we arrived back in Baton Rouge to move in with my parents and start our new life in August 2016. The news called it a 500-year flood. Eight months of living with my parents. Eight months of watching my mom's mind slip away, day by day. We gave up the idea of finding our own place. How could we abandon my father to face this alone?

Mom has "Mean Alzheimer's." Jimmy's dad had "Quiet Alzheimer's." I want my mother to slip into Quiet Alzheimer's.

Mom thinks she is fine. She hates my dad. She hates her life. She hates me. Restless, she must be entertained like a two-year-old. Every hour she asks, "What are we going to do now?" It's exhausting. I want to crawl into bed and not wake up. Some days, I think she does too.

When the floodwater finally receded, I tried my 2.3-mile neighborhood loop, but the bridge over the dam had been swept away. The broken pieces leaned against the bamboo, the sidewalk smeared with foul, sticky mud. My beautiful trail was devastated.

I felt like that broken bridge. Everything I knew washed away. My shattered life propped up by thin reeds of bamboo, ready to snap.

Could I be built anew? I didn't think so. Pieces of me seemed to dissolve every day. It would take time to sort out the next steps.

Without the lake, walking the neighborhood felt monotonous and dull. The lake that had given me comfort was in limbo, but I trusted nature to nudge it back to life. That faith gave me hope.

"The bridge is back," Dad announced two months later while I fixed dinner. He'd sweet-talked Mom into a walk, and they had discovered the rebuilt bridge.

The next morning, I woke up early and practically skipped to the path. As the trail turned, the new footbridge beckoned me back to my routine: across the dam, past the swings and slides, through the neighborhood to the smaller bridge and home. I did a little victory dance and shouted, "Whoo-hoo!"

The lake is a gift. My walks are meditation. They clear my head and wake up my spirit. My body feels heavy these days. Comfort eating leaves me with sugar hangovers and creeping weight. In Los Angeles three years ago, I lost a bunch of weight, and I felt proud. Now I'm pulling larger sizes from the closet. But at the lake, I feel fit, free, and light on my feet. The elephant lifts from my chest. I finish by stretching on the back-deck railing. Morning sun pours through the giant oaks, and I lift my eyes into the warmth. Gratitude soaks through my skin and seeps into my heart.

A few days later, I see my White Heron again. He stares into the water, then—flash—his head darts under. He rises with a fish, still and efficient, and eats.

OK, I get it. Stand and be still. Just be. You don't have to figure it all out today, Peggy. Just be.

Then he takes flight, giant wings crossing right in front of me, over the bridge, circling the lake. He doesn't just fly—he soars. Effortless. Free. Graceful.

I feel the promise and blessing of my beautiful White Heron, my spirit guide.

I return to my rhythm, walking several times a week. I miss my L.A. walking buddies. I need a Baton Rouge walking buddy—someone to walk this tough life with me.

Across the street are our neighbors, Alice and Bobby. Every April, they throw a crawfish boil—The Crawfish Extravaganza. I've seen the clever invitations on my parents' counter for years.

"My friend Alice lives there," my friend Vanda said recently, pointing. "She has a great crawfish boil. You should go."

"I would love to."

When Dad brings in the invitation in mid-April, I announce, "I want to go this year!"

The day arrives, and I freeze at the upstairs window. I haven't been in the mood to meet new people. We socialize with family and old friends, but even that feels exhausting. Beneath my smile, I feel like a fraud. The minute we step back inside, reality hits. The Big A waits.

Cars snake around the circle looking for spots. People carry covered dishes, cases of beer, and bottles of wine. I fetch the mail, hear live music in the backyard, smell the boil. A "Cajun Crawfish Boil" truck hisses in their driveway, a huge pot rolling over fire.

"That's it," I say out loud. "I'm going." Jimmy is golfing. My parents are with one of my sisters. I'm going solo.

I pull on a blue-and-white top and white shorts, sunscreen, red lipstick, cute sandals, and a straw hat. I feel like I'm crashing a party—and I'm thrilled.

I knock. No answer. Through the glass, I see the crowd in back. I open the door and step into a lovely living room; the dining table to the left is piled with cakes, cookies, brownies, fruit salad—an altar of sugar.

"Is Alice here?" I ask a woman at the sink.

"She's outside in the red shirt," she says.

I take a breath and head out, blurting, "Hi, Alice. I'm Peggy—my parents are your neighbors, Myles and Sherry. They couldn't come, but I wanted to meet you."

"I'm so glad you did!" she beams, the perfect Southern hostess. She introduces me to her pretty daughter, Tricia, and adorable granddaughters, Izzy and Maddie, sitting poolside with their legs in the water. A giant blow-up crawfish floats by as Alice points me toward the boiled crawfish. Aluminum buckets brim with spicy red tails, corn, and potatoes on red-and-white checked tables under white tents and sunflowers in vases. I sit and dig in. The juices run to my elbows; I'm grateful for the sleeveless top. Paper towels bloom around my little mountain of shells. My nose runs. My mouth burns. I chug a blessedly cold Barq's Root Beer.

"Hi, I'm Peggy. I live across the street," I tell the couple at my table. They share their long friendship with Alice and Bobby. Another couple met them on a music cruise and drove from Florida yesterday. I met our sweet neighbors, Pete and Karen.

"We know your lovely parents," Karen says. "Don't miss the food on the other side of the pool. Bobby's an excellent Cajun chef."

"And my wife's homemade chocolate cake," Pete adds.

By the grill, two guys charbroil oysters—garlic, lemon, butter—Parmesan melting on top. They smell like heaven. Bobby, charming and bayou-born, smiles.

"I'm glad you came," he says. "The boiled crawfish are just the appetizer. Get a bowl of my crawfish stew and the famous shrimp salad."

This is my kind of party. I snapped a photo of the oysters and text Jimmy: *Meet me at the crawfish boil. Amazing!*

Wow! Charbroiled oysters? Can I come in my golf shirt, or should I shower?

It's a crawfish boil. Throw on some deodorant.

By the pool, I recognize a woman—Maxine—from a Blues Foundation event. Within minutes, we discover we share a birthday, July 21. Birthday twins. Instant connection. We exchange numbers and promise a joint brunch.

Vanda arrives just as Jimmy strides in from across the street. She's a spark of Brazilian fire, and we adore her.

Bands rotate all afternoon, and we dance on the patio. Jimmy and I wander to the dock and sit in Adirondack chairs.

He lights a cigar. The lake sparkles. It is heavenly. For the first time in a long time, I realized I hadn't thought about Mom all afternoon.

"Thank you for having us—what a party," I tell Alice as we leave at seven. Five hours of Louisiana joy. Just what the doctor ordered.

"Alice, would you like to walk with me sometime? I'm looking for a walking buddy," I hear myself say.

"I'd love to," she says, and we swap numbers.

Soon we're meeting early to circle the lake. Alice and Bobby fold us into their life—LSU games with extra season tickets, dancing at a local bar, and a dinner party with Bobby's band. They include my parents. Mom loves music and she is clapping, singing, smiling. Everyone knows she has Alzheimer's; everyone is kind. Alice brings Dad wine. Bobby jitterbugs with Mom in the living room. For an evening, she is alive and vibrant. We walked home at eleven. I'm stunned my parents have lasted this long.

"I thought y'all would have left hours ago," I tease.

"Well, your mom was having so much fun," Dad says. "And it's not like we had to drive across town."

"Have you seen Big Blue?" Alice asks one morning. "He's a Blue Heron. He's been on our deck."

"No, not yet."

A week later, we cross the bridge, and there he stands on a log among turtles—slate-blue feathers, long, sharp beak. Strong and proud. We tiptoe to the midpoint, and I snapped a photo. He doesn't notice us. We slip away, blessed by Big Blue. I realize how special it is that Alice shared him with me. In Alice, I found a friend. In that moment, I felt the healing of nature.

That night, I looked up the Blue Heron: the ability to progress and evolve; innate wisdom to navigate life and co-create your circumstances.

"Am I progressing? Am I evolving?" I ask Jimmy. "I put it into the universe to find a walking buddy, and Alice appeared."

"I'm proud of you," he says. "You're a good daughter. Your dad appreciates us being here."

One evening, we coax Mom to take a stroll to the lake. The humidity is kind—rare for Louisiana. A soft breeze rustles Spanish moss with angelic pastel clouds reflecting on the water. We sit on a bench and watch a gaggle of Canadian

Geese waddle down the path and slip into the lake. Six fuzzy goslings trail their mother in a straight line.

"Look how precious," Mom says.

"Adorable. Let's swing."

"Really?"

"Yes, Mom. It'll be fun." She laughs as I lift her from the bench, and we head for the swings. Soon we're soaring. Dad watches, smiling. We giggle like two little girls. For ten minutes, I forgot her Alzheimer's.

Memory rises like a tide: five years old, piling into the blue station wagon with the Jackson family for a picnic at the local park and running to the swings while Mom and Aunt Margaret spread a tablecloth, bologna sandwiches, potato chips, and bright red Kool-Aid in Dixie cups. Life is simple, carefree, and full of promises. After lunch, we would scale the grandstand, and I would dance, a star on a big stage.

"I'm ready to go home now," Mom says, dragging her feet and hopping off. The moment on the swings leaves me light, serenity blooming in my chest. The sunset is breathtaking. I feel blessed.

Before we go, I have Mom and Dad sit on the bench again. "Look at each other and act like you love each other,"

I joke, snapping photos. "Now kiss." They giggle and oblige like teenagers. The lighting is perfect. Walking back, they hold hands while I post the pictures with #truelove.

At home, Dad pours himself a white wine, iced tea for Mom, and they settle in with the news. I throw together dinner: a deli roasted chicken, a bagged salad brightened with tomato, avocado, cucumber, steamed baby carrots, and rolls warmed in the oven. I cook now; Jimmy handles cleanup. We have our evening rhythm.

While the chicken warms, I Google the spiritual meaning of Canadian Geese: bravery, loyalty (never leaving one behind), teamwork, confidence, protection, fellowship, communication, and determination. Simple words—another shot in the arm. More crumbs to light the path.

The White Heron, the Blue Heron, and the Canadian Geese have taught me the lessons of the lake—the gifts of coming home and being here for Mom and Dad. Sometimes I must stand still; sometimes I have to plunge my head into the water and grope for a clue. Other times, I waddle along the edges or release control and let the current take me where it will. Maybe one day I will fly again. But today, right now—the lesson is simple: Keep moving forward.

Louisiana Charbroiled Oysters

Ingredients for the Sauce:

1 stick unsalted butter, room temperature - very soft
1 pinch Kosher salt
½ tsp. Paprika
1 tsp. freshly ground black pepper
3 cloves of garlic, minced or grated
4 Tbsp. Pecorino Romano cheese, grated
1 pinch of cayenne
1 pinch of white pepper
Juice of ½ of a lemon
1 tsp. Italian parsley, minced

Instructions for the Sauce:

Whisk together all ingredients. Set Aside.

Ingredients for the Oysters:

1 dozen large freshly shucked Louisiana oysters on the half shell
Oyster Sauce, above
¾ cup of Pecorino Romano cheese, grated
Minced Italian parsley to garnish
Hot French bread
Lemon wedges

Instructions for the Oysters:

Heat a charcoal or gas grill until it reaches extremely high temperatures.
Place the oysters on the hottest spot on the grill and let them cook in their juices for a few minutes, just until they start to bubble and the edges curl.

Top each with a generous portion of the sauce, enough to fill up the shell.

When the sauce bubbles and sizzles, sprinkle each oyster with a generous amount of Pecorino Romano cheese.

Let the oysters grill until the sauce on the edges of the shells gets nice and brown. Larger oysters may take another minute.

Garnish with minced parsley.

Serve while sizzling with lemon wedges and hot French bread to soak up the butter sauce.

Yield:

Serves four as an appetizer (3 oysters each)

Notes:

Once you have tried charbroiled oysters, you'll never want to eat them any other way—the best part is dipping the French Bread in the juices left behind after you have eaten the oysters.

CHAPTER SIX
BEST FRIENDS

"Let's take a girls' weekend trip with our mothers," my "cousin" Stephanie suggests.

We are eating lunch with Mom, Dad, and Stephanie's mother, whom I have always called Aunt Rita. We sit at a large booth at City Cafe, our neighborhood joint. Shrimp poboys and grilled oysters fill the table. Stephanie and Aunt Rita have driven in from New Orleans for the day.

Aunt Rita is my mom's oldest and dearest friend. They both attended Catholic school and have known each other since kindergarten. They grew up side by side in the Irish Channel of New Orleans, in the St. Thomas housing project built in the '30s for working-class families. The two-story units had a small living room and kitchen, three tiny bedrooms upstairs, a front porch, and a fenced yard. Between the buildings stretched a communal green dotted with oak trees.

I remember visiting my grandparents there as a child —picking acorns, making forts in the bushes, feeling part of a lively community of Irish, Italian, and Cajun families who all knew each other.

For as long as I can remember, Aunt Rita and Stephanie have been part of our family. Stephanie, just a year older than me and my mother's goddaughter, was the big sister I never had. Pretty with short brown hair, big brown eyes, and a warm smile, she was smart, athletic, and fun-loving. Mom adored her. Every summer, she'd spend a week with us, staying up late, bonding over our Barbies, books, and records. Even now, Stephanie makes Mom feel extra special with gifts, cards, and visits. Since Mom's diagnosis with the Big A, Stephanie has made an effort to bring Aunt Rita to visit.

Aunt Rita herself is a force—sharp, funny, blunt, and colorful. She and Uncle Rock raised their six kids in uptown New Orleans. She has a dry sense of humor and a colorful personality. She tells you like it is! With Mom, she forms half of a legendary duo—two lifelong friends whose escapades with their childhood crew (Barbara, Althea, and

Net) could fill a book. Time has taken Althea, and Net, and Barbara now lives in Missouri. But Rita remains. Together, she and Mom light up any room. Spending time with them is always filled with lots of laughs and stories.

"Where should we go?" I ask Stephanie, and we brainstorm places while Aunt Rita and Mom chit-chat with my dad. Well, Aunt Rita and Dad chit-chat. Mom has been quiet in social situations lately.

"How about Natchez?" Stephanie suggests.

"Perfect," I reply, telling her places to stay and fun things to do.

The following month, Stephanie and Aunt Rita drove to Baton Rouge to spend the night with us on Friday night. On Saturday morning, we pack the car with snacks, bottled water, and magazines and head the ninety miles north to Natchez. We have booked two double rooms at the Natchez Grand Hotel overlooking the Mississippi River. I had hosted a cultural weekend tour to Natchez the year before, so I know the sights and have a list ready. And my friend, chef and author Regina Charboneau, has opened a new restaurant, King's Tavern, which I am eager to try.

"Where are we going?" Mom asks as we pull onto the interstate.

"Natchez," Aunt Rita answers smoothly.

"Oh, that's right," Mom says, embarrassed to have forgotten.

We roll past the Baton Rouge airport into the Tunica Hills area of Louisiana, passing plantations and the quaint town of St. Francisville, then cross into Mississippi. I suggest lunch options—The Pig Out Barbeque or Mama's Tamales. At the mention of tamales, Mom perks up.

"I remember going with my dad on the streetcar to buy tamales from the Tamale Man's cart on the corner of St. Charles and Napoleon. He'd wrap a dozen tamales in a newspaper, and they would still be warm when we got home. We would each get three tamales, but it was never enough. I could eat a dozen myself!" she laughs. We all laugh along with her, relishing her talkative nature and the way she shares her memories.

"I remember those tamales as a kid. Mom, remember when I brought the wonderful tamales home from Los Angeles?" I said.

"Yes, those were the best!" she replied. I'm surprised she remembers.

A work friend in L.A. made them with her family every year for Christmas, and she would take orders, $1.00 a tamale. I ordered four dozen, froze them, wrapped them up in newspaper, stuck them in a large zip-lock plastic bag, then placed them in my suitcase between sweaters and scarves as we flew home to Louisiana for the holidays. They were still frozen when we arrived in Baton Rouge.

The next night, my sisters and their families came over to my parents' house. Mom and I cooked a big pot of chili to serve with the tamales and topped them with cheese and chopped onions. The tamales were a massive hit with my family. Unfortunately, I changed jobs the following year, and tamale night didn't become a Sweeney holiday food tradition.

My friend Scott brought some tamales back to Los Angeles from his family's Christmas vacation a few years later. His mother, Betty, grew up in Mexico, and they would make tamales with his aunts every year. My parents were coming to visit us that year, right after Christmas, and Scott invited us over for tamales. I told Scott that Mom and I would make chili to serve with his tamales.

"I have never eaten tamales with chili," he said dramatically. He is a bit of a diva!

"You have no idea what you are missing! Tamales with homemade chili, grated cheese, and chopped onions with a dollop of sour cream on top are one of my all-time favorite meals." I told him. Sure enough, they loved it!

"Now I want some tamales!" Mom says.

"Me too," Aunt Rita chimes in, and we all giggle. For a moment, it feels like old times.

"What is that?" Aunt Rita asks as we pass a whimsical pink building shaped like a woman in a ballgown.

"Oh, that's a famous diner," I reply.

"Let's go there for lunch," Stephanie decides, making a quick U-turn and pulling into the parking lot. Aunt Rita and Mom squeal with delight in the back seat.

"This is cute," Mom says. "What is it?"

"A lovely little cafe, Mom."

"The front door is at the bottom of the skirt of her dress. Now that takes the cake," Aunt Rita says.

"This is a great idea. It's a little early for lunch, but it smells great," Stephanie says as we walk through the front entrance, a gift shop selling homemade jams and jellies in Mason jars, honey, and candles.

"Y'all can sit wherever you would like," a sassy waitress holding a tray of delicious-looking slices of pie tells us.

We find a table for four in the middle of the dining room, and she soon comes over to hand us menus. Stephanie has a huge, sweet tooth and goes directly to the dessert section in the back to peruse the pie selection.

"Did y'all see the pie? We will get pie for dessert!" she announces.

Mom, Aunt Rita, and I ordered chicken salad sandwiches with a cup of homemade chicken noodle soup. Stephanie orders a grilled chicken salad, saving her calories since she wants pie. The great pie debate begins–lemon meringue, chocolate meringue, pecan, banana cream?

"What kind of pie did you get?" Aunt Rita asks an older couple at the next table.

"Lemon meringue and pecan. Both were great," the woman says.

"We should all get a different slice to share," Stephanie says.

"No, that's crazy! Let's just get two slices and split them since we will be eating at Chef Regina's restaurant tonight, and you will want her famous biscuits and dessert. Plus, we have to get Darby's Fudge later," I say.

"Fudge? You didn't tell me about the fudge," Stephanie exclaims. We settled on a slice of lemon meringue and chocolate meringue.

The waitress brings us delicious, sweet tea and our lunch, but we can't wait to get the pie.

"I have to go to the bathroom," Mom says.

"I need to go too," Aunt Rita says, and off they go.

"Nanny seems good today. She doesn't have that blank look she had this morning." Stephanie says.

"I haven't seen her this animated in weeks. It's because y'all are here. Thanks for making this happen. She needs her friends. She needs your mom and you."

"Peggy, come here," Aunt Rita calls me from the bathroom hallway. *Oh no*, I think. *This can't be good*. I jump up and head to the bathroom.

I find them doubled over laughing as the ladies' bathroom is a single room with two toilets sitting side by side with no divider.

"The friends who pee together stay together!" I quip and we howl with laughter. I snap a picture with my iPhone.

They are like little girls giggling over a secret joke. Back at our table, the pie has arrived. Stephanie is already taking a bite.

"What's going on back there?" she asks. She and everyone else in the diner heard us laughing. I gave her the scoop and showed her the picture. She jumps up and heads to the bathroom. She is not missing this silliness!

Stephanie comes back with both of them trailing behind her, laughing hysterically. I'm now eating a big bite of lemon pie.

"Y'all better sit down and get some pie while you can!" I say.

"You weren't supposed to start dessert without us," Aunt Rita says.

They sit and join me as we attack the pie with great enthusiasm—forks crossing like swords, fighting for crumbs.

"Best pie ever!" I declare.

"Do you want to lick the plate?" Mom teases, laughing.

"We should stop by on the way back tomorrow and get some pies to take home," Stephanie says.

"It's not open on Sunday."

"Damn!" she replies.

"Y'all didn't like that pie, did you?" the waitress says as she hands us the bill and clears the table.

"No, we hated it!" Mom jokes, smiling at the waitress.

Stephanie grabs the check.

"My treat. A late birthday lunch for Nanny."

Before heading to the car, we stopped in the gift shop and bought a small Mason jar of local honey wrapped in burlap, tied with twine. Pulling out of the parking lot, we are still laughing about the bathroom with two toilets. Mom is glowing with delight. Aunt Rita and Stephanie are a shot in the arm for both of us. It feels so good to be having fun again! We are only ten miles from Natchez. I pull up the GPS on my phone to find our way to downtown Natchez.

"Let's stop at Darby's on Main Street," I direct Stephanie once we get into the Natchez city limits. I point out Mama's Tamales and the Pig Out Barbeque restaurants, where we almost had lunch.

"I'm glad we ate at our place," Aunt Rita says.

"Where?" Mom asks.

"The Cupboard, the cute diner where we just had lunch, and the great pies," I say.

"I didn't go there," she says. Stephanie and I look at each other.

"Well, we can take you next time, Nanny," Stephanie tells her.

"Yes, next time, Sherry," Aunt Rita repeats, and the car falls silent.

The dreaded silence of acceptance catches our breath, weighs on our hearts, and calcifies in our bones. They are surrendering to the truth of Mom's Alzheimer's.

One minute, Mom seems fine, and you forget about the Big A. But a minute or an hour later, it all falls apart. The truth slaps you in the face, and it will never be the same. You lose hope. Everyone has been in denial, even after learning of her official diagnosis. I know what is going through their minds and feel for them. It's not easy to process emotionally. I look over at Stephanie, and she has tears rolling down her face.

"This town is so cute," Aunt Rita says as we pass block after block of colorful Victorian homes and make our way downtown.

Within minutes, we are in front of Darby's Gift Shop. I'm grateful for the distraction and know that a dip into Darby's will put a smile on our faces. It is a fabulous gift shop owned by Darby and her husband. The store is the heart and pulse of downtown Natchez. Initially, they made and sold crafts at festivals and then opened their store, which has continued to expand through the years. They now own this store and Darby's Furniture and Accessories stores across the street.

The gift shop is in a beautiful historical building, filled with everything you can imagine: clothing, candles, wreaths, jewelry, shoes, gifts, cookware, jams, bottles of flavorings, seasonings, cookbooks, flags, decorative signs, and Christmas ornaments. But the primary focus is their homemade fudge that greets you as you enter the door with the intoxicating smell. Flavor after mouthwatering flavor, deliciously displayed behind a sparkling glass counter in front of the cash register. Behind the cash register is another counter with a huge mixing bowl; if you time it right, someone is making a giant batch of fudge right in front of you. They ship it year-round across the globe, and sales are huge during the holidays. Once you've tried Darby's fudge, you'll never want to buy it from anywhere else. It is the best fudge ever!

Within minutes, Mom and Aunt Rita are standing at the counter, sampling the flavors on tiny tasting spoons.

"This is delicious. I want to get some for Dad," Mom says as she tries the Butterfinger flavor.

"Try this one. It's Cookies and Cream," Aunt Rita says, sticking out her tiny spoon for Mom to taste.

"My favorite is pumpkin spice! What kind do you think Dad would like?" I ask Mom as I stand there licking my pumpkin sample.

I request another sample from the sweet young girl behind the counter. She hands me another spoon with my other favorite, Peanut Butter, with a layer of chocolate.

"Stephanie, come try this!"

"I'm still full from the pie!" she says, laughing, but then tries it and asks to try the praline flavor.

We all ooh and aah over the fudge, then meander our way through the store.

I found cute earrings and a fun red tunic top perfect for Christmas afternoon with my red cowboy boots. Darby arrives, and I hug her and then introduce her. She is beautiful and welcoming. Everyone loves Darby. Mom leans down to pet Maggie, their black lab. She is the store mascot and always sits by the front door.

"She's so cute. I'm tired," she says.

"Alright, we are leaving, Mom. Let's go check into the hotel," I say.

Aunt Rita holds Mom's hand, and they clutch their little red and gold fudge boxes tied with gold ribbon. We load into the car with our packages and turn down the street to the Grand Hotel at the end of the road. Unfortunately, we can't get adjoining rooms, but we are down the hall from each other.

"Do you want to go for a walk?" Stephanie asks me as we get off the elevator. "Mom can come to your room and stay with Nanny," she whispers, knowing I can't leave Mom alone.

Once in our room, Mom goes to the bathroom while I change into sweats and sneakers. The weather is sunny and crisp, a perfect fall day. I'm excited to show Stephanie the walk along the bluffs overlooking the Mississippi River.

"Where's Dad? I want to give him his fudge," Mom says as she comes out of the bathroom.

"He's at home in Baton Rouge."

"Can we go see him?"

"No, Mom, we are spending the night here. We will see him tomorrow when we go home." She looks sad and lost, and it breaks my heart.

"I miss him," she says, looking like she is going to cry.

I pull out my phone and called Dad. "Mom wants to talk to you," and I handed her the phone.

"Where are you?" she asks him.

"I'm home working. Are y'all having a good time?"

"Yes, I bought some fudge for you!" she tells him. "I love you. Bye," and she hands me the phone. The talk with Dad seemed to soothe her. Still, the truth sits heavy: Mom struggles when she is away from Dad, even though she argues with him constantly.

Soon, Mom and Aunt Rita are relaxing on the two double beds, watching *Ellen*.

"Y'all have a good time. We'll be fine," Aunt Rita says.

Stephanie and I walked along the gorgeous Bluff Trail, grateful to be alone and to catch up without our mothers. Natchez never gets old. It is the off-season, and it is quiet. We continued down the inclined street to the "Under the River" area of Natchez, which has several restaurants, including the famous Magnolia Cafe. We strolled past the gorgeous Rosalie Plantation, surrounded by 400-year-old Oak trees, then through downtown Natchez. The Greek Revival buildings are old and stately, remnants of a bygone era.

She fills me in on her husband, Chuck, and her grown son, Wayne. I tell her the latest with Mom and how it affects Dad and me. I tell her how strong Jimmy is for me.

"It's getting harder. I'm not built to be a caregiver. I'm no good at this. I have no patience."

"You are doing the best you can. I know it's hard. I can't believe how Nanny is slipping away like this. She seems confused and not like the Nanny I know. I think this trip is good for her, being with Mom. I'm glad we did this." Stephanie tells me.

"This trip is good for me, too! I can't believe we haven't done this before," I say, hugging her.

"Maybe we can do another trip in the spring," she says.

"Maybe, I hope so," but I know deep down this is the first and last girls' trip we will ever do with our mothers.

We look out at the Mississippi River and the bridge that crosses over to Vidalia, Louisiana, as the sun begins to go down. The color of the Mighty Mississippi is dark, muddy, and mysterious, but the river is magnificent, with the sun glistening on it.

That night we dined at King's Tavern. It is the oldest standing building in Mississippi and is reported to be haunted. My dear friend, Regina, and her husband, Doug, own the restaurant and the Charboneau Rum Distillery next door. Their youngest son, Jean Luc, is bartending that night and tells me his parents will be there soon.

The restaurant is rustic, and we sit at a large wooden table with benches. We order the most delicious appetizers, salads, and Regina's famous brisket, cooked over several days in an incredible sauce that melts in your mouth. It is truly a culinary experience.

Regina and Doug arrive while we eat and greet us at our table. I see her and jump up excitedly to hug them. They are gracious hosts. Regina sits with us and tells us the history of the restaurant. Jean Luc comes over to our table to tell us the ghost stories and even shows us a video on his phone of a ghost that appeared on their video security cameras. They are enchanting. Mom, Aunt Rita, and Stephanie are impressed with the VIP treatment and Regina's southern hospitality. We enjoy every minute.

Mom loves everything. We eat well and are sopping up every drop of the brisket gravy with Regina's world-famous biscuits.

"Seriously, Regina, I could eat just a bowl of your brisket gravy with a basket of your hot buttered biscuits!" I say.

"You are too kind," she says graciously, sending us her heavenly desserts—Bread Pudding and Natchez Pecan Pie. You can never go wrong with a meal from Chef Regina. Her cookbooks are gorgeous, featuring delicious recipes accompanied by stunning pictures, displayed in her formal dining room, verandah, or back patio. Before we leave, we go upstairs to the restaurant gift shop and purchase her jams and jellies. I give Regina one last hug. For a few hours, we were wrapped in warmth and laughter.

"Y'all want to go to the Casino?" I ask as we get in the car. But everyone is tired, so we head back to our hotel rooms. Mom brushes her teeth and then climbs into bed, still wearing her clothes.

"Mom, I packed your nightgown."

"That's okay. I'm more comfortable like this."

I let it go and called Dad so she could tell him goodnight.

"Did you have a nice time? It sounds like you had a great dinner at Regina's restaurant. They are such nice people." His voice is deep and loud, so I can hear him talking across the room when he is on the phone with her.

"It was wonderful! Where are you?" she says, smiling.

"I'm home. I'll see you tomorrow. Goodnight."

I turn the lights out and soon hear my mother snoring lightly.

Through thick and thin, Mom and Aunt Rita have been there for each other, and seventy-five years of friendship is etched in memory if not always in mind. They are role models for what it means to show up, to laugh, and to endure.

Having Stephanie by my side warms my heart, knowing I can rely on her and share my struggles. This girls' trip was a special treat for all of us. As my mom's mind slowly fades away and I trudge through life in the A-Zone, I

112

will hold tight to these moments: the smiles, the laughter, the shopping, the dinner, and the crazy cafe lunch.

Life is short. Eat the pie and savor the sweetness of every crumb of happiness with your best friends!

Mom's Lemon Icebox Pie

Ingredients:

5 egg whites
2 Tbsp. sugar
1 can of condensed milk
1 Tbsp. of grated lemon peel
½ cup lemon juice
1 Graham Cracker Crust
Whipped Cream or Cool Whip

Instructions:

Grate one tablespoon of lemon peel and spread on the Graham cracker crust.
Beat egg whites until very stiff, add sugar gradually.
In a separate bowl, mix the condensed milk and lemon juice. Mix well.
Fold into the stiffly beaten egg whites.
Pour mixture into the crust and refrigerate until ready to serve.
Add Whipped Cream or Cool Whip before serving.

Yield:

Serves 8

Family Notes:

Once a month, my mother would pray the rosary with a group of women friends at Miss Helen's house. I remember Miss Helen had a statue of the Virgin Mary on her front lawn and was very religious. The women would bring sandwiches, casseroles, and desserts for a social lunch after the rosary. My mother wasn't a baker, but I remember her making this pie for the rosary. I think she found the recipe in our local newspaper. It was a hit, and soon she made it for us for Easter dinner, and it made it into our family cookbook. In the summer, the kids were invited to join the rosary and enjoy a yummy lunch afterward. I obediently said the rosary along with the women, but my mind drifted to the sumptuous lunch to come, especially my mom's pie!

CHAPTER SEVEN
THE FASHION SHOW

I drink my black coffee in the living room, reading my inspirational prayer and meditation books. I'm grateful for the morning "me time" before everyone else wakes up. I hear the main bedroom door open and close, then a shuffle down the hall. I'm waiting for today's fashion show. Here she comes.

My mother steps into the living room dressed in the mix-matched outfit she has selected for today—navy blue pants inside out, a black and white checked top, a metallic gold sweater coat, and of course, the purse.

She carries the old black purse everywhere she goes, even in the house. It overflows with brushes, socks, winter gloves, rosary beads, half-eaten candy bars, angels, lipsticks, powder, eyeshadow, and anything else she may need for the day. Last Christmas, I bought her a beautiful new black handbag, and she loved it on Christmas morning. I transferred all her belongings into it, but days later, she was back to her old purse. The new one is now in my closet. One day, I may use it. Maybe.

She shuffles across the room and sits next to me on the sofa, all dolled up. The blank stare is the cherry on top.

"Good morning, Mom."

Don't say anything about her outfit. I tell myself. It's not worth the fight.

My nieces will be embarrassed if she shows up at Grandparents' Day dressed like this.

She isn't my mother anymore. She was always beautifully dressed and perfectly matched, like most Southern women. Her closet is filled with lovely clothes, with boxes of shoes and purses lined neatly on the top shelf. Now she wears the same clothes over and over, in odd combinations—sometimes she wears the same clothes for days at a time.

She sleeps in her clothes. I tried to encourage her to wear her pretty nightgowns to bed, but she refused, so I gave up. Her matching gowns and robes now hang untouched in her closet, collecting dust.

For our "girls only," Royal Wedding watch breakfast, my youngest sister, Kelly, gave her the cutest pink-and-white striped Kate Spade pajamas with matching slippers and a pink and white fascinator hat. We woke up at 5:30 a.m. and drove to our friend Kathryn's house for 6:30. Kathryn, the "hostess with the mostess" served shrimp and grits with homemade biscuits. Mimosas and champagne flowed throughout the celebration. For dessert, we enjoyed a small wedding cake with buttercream frosting and raspberries.

We laughed and cried watching the beautiful wedding. In her pretty PJs, Mom loved every minute. The local paper sent a reporter and a photographer to cover the party for the society section. The newspaper clipping sits in my bedroom, and the pretty pajamas now hang in her closet—cherished memories of a special day.

Kelly recently told me she'd like the pajamas back if Mom isn't going to wear them. I wanted to snag them, but then I remembered they needed ironing. I don't have the energy or the patience for that.

"What are we doing today?" Mom asks.

"It's Grandparents' Day at St. George for Izzy and Jillian."

"Is it time to go?"

"Not quite, Mom," I glance at the cable box clock. It's only 7:30 a.m., and the program begins at 10:30. How will we fill the next hours? This is why they call a day with an Alzheimer's patient a thirty-six-hour day. At least we have somewhere to go today. The worst days are the empty ones.

I walk to the kitchen and pour her coffee in a pink ceramic cup, the last one left from the pink China set she had years ago. I add powdered cream and sugar to her coffee, shaking my head. Recently, I asked her when she started drinking it that way.

"I never drank black coffee," she says defensively, and I drop the subject.

Mom always took her coffee black. I find it strange, I told Jimmy later that night as we brushed our teeth, side by side.

"I remember her staying up late at night watching Johnny Carson, smoking her daily cigarette, and drinking black microwaved coffee leftover from breakfast," he says, laughing.

Early in our marriage, Jimmy and my mother were night owls together. Whenever we visited, they would stay up watching late-night television, drinking coffee, and smoking long after Dad and I went to bed. It was their bonding time. She loved Jimmy's New York smartass sense of humor and his off-color language. Jimmy was the one who taught her to curse, shocking us all.

She quit smoking cigarettes years ago, and Jimmy soon followed—except for his daily cigar. I suppose she gave up black coffee, too. How did I miss it?

"I can't find my lipsticks, Peggy, did you take them?"

She digs through her purse. She asks the same question every day, convinced I'm stealing from her. Once, Jimmy found her rummaging through our dresser drawers. When he offered to help, she just stared at him blankly and walked away.

I set her coffee down and leaned over to hug her, noticing her eyebrows drawn with a red marker. Where did that come from?

"No, Mom, I don't have your lipsticks, but I'm sure we can find them. Let's go fix your hair and make-up."

"No, I don't need you to help me. I already did my own."

Defeated, I walked to the kitchen. I've stopped asking if she is hungry. I prepare breakfast and bring it to her, hoping she will eat a few bites. She is losing weight. Her clothes are starting to hang on her small frame. Sweets are the only thing she seems to crave.

I pull out frozen waffles, butter, blueberry jam, and an overripe banana. I'm grateful to be able to do this small task. The waffle pops up too soon, so I toast it again. We like our waffles golden brown. As I butter her waffle, I toast two more for me. I spread the jam, add slices of banana on the side, and then cut the waffle into bite-sized pieces like you would for a child. I pull out a tray from the top of the refrigerator. I pour orange juice into a small cocktail glass. I wish we still had the cute juice glasses we grew up with back in the '60s. Maybe it would trigger a memory. I love it when she tells me old stories, and I marvel that her brain can remember the past so vividly, yet not even five minutes ago.

Taking her meds out of the daily medicine case, I place them in a tiny bowl on the tray. Maybe she will take them; maybe she won't. It's a crapshoot. We sometimes find the pills in the sofa cushions, inside magazines, in her bathroom drawers, on the floor, or even in the garbage can.

"Mom, you have to take your pills! Why are you throwing them away?"

"I didn't throw them away. You take them!"

It always escalates. One day, maybe I'll stop fighting. The pills aren't helping anyway. She isn't getting better. So, what's the point?

I carry our breakfast to the living room and put the tray on her lap. She takes a bite and thanks me. I take my plate off the tray, sit on the sofa next to her, and dig in. One waffle for her. Two for me. We watched the *Today Show* and eat our waffles in silence. I never knew a frozen waffle could taste so good. The days of protein drinks and morning power walks are rare now. Give me carbs, fat, and sugar. They are my consolation prize for caregiving.

Today, she takes her pills without protest—a small victory. I cling to those. I look for little victories every day.

The struggles remind me I'm not good at this. I'm not good at mothering my mother. I miss being a daughter and having my mother take care of me. I want to wake up and find her cooking breakfast for me in the kitchen. I crave the fried egg in the hole she made for us as children. I want to sit with my little sisters at our old kitchen table and dip the rounded-out butter-fried piece of bread in the hot, runny egg yolk. I want to hear her laughter. I wanted to feel her energy as she buzzed around the kitchen. I want to experience her zest for life again, even for a moment. I want to feel my Mama's love. I need to feel my Mama's love desperately.

I wonder when I started calling her Mom instead of Mama. I've noticed that my three sisters now call her Mom too. We always called her Mama. Did that change as we got older, or did it change when she became someone we no longer recognize?

I know my Mama is still there. I want to find her again. I want to scream, "Come back, please! I need you."

I need her to help me navigate this journey. I'm falling daily. I want her to go to her well-stocked medicine cabinet and put a Band-Aid on my emotional scrapes and burns, but there isn't one big enough to put over my aching heart.

"It's time to go. We are going to be late!" she says. The anxiety is building for her and me. This will be her mantra for the next two hours. I look down and notice she has two different shoes on—one orange flat shoe and a black loafer. I strategize in my head for ways to convince her to change clothes and shoes before we leave without a fight.

I say the Serenity Prayer in my head. *God, grant me the serenity to accept the things I cannot change—the courage to change the things I can and the wisdom to know the difference.* The problem is, I don't know what I can change. Each day is different, and I have no courage, no wisdom. I feel hopeless and empty as I walk back to the kitchen with the tray. I stuff the rest of her waffle into my mouth, drag my finger across the plate for the leftover blueberry jam, and lick the dredges off my finger. Sugar is a pacifier for my pain.

"Mom, do you want to color?"

"Sure"

We sit at the kitchen table and begin coloring in adult coloring books. We love it. It passes the time. You don't have to think. It's a coloring meditation. We have a large plastic zip-lock bag containing markers and another bag with crayons. She is much better at coloring than I am. She stays in the lines. She takes her time. The sun pours through the kitchen blinds, and we work side by side diligently, coloring our pictures of flowers. Whoever had the brilliant idea of adult coloring books must have had a parent with Alzheimer's. I have another adult coloring book with scenes of New York. I don't know where it is now. It disappeared with her makeup. A few weeks ago, I colored a taxicab, and she colored a hot dog stand. It made me want to go back to New York for happier times.

"Sherry, are you ready to go?" Dad says as he comes into the kitchen.

"Where are we going?"

"Grandparents Day"

"Oh, that's right."

"Mom, let's go get dressed," I chirp, and miraculously, she follows me to the bedroom. She allows me to help her change into another outfit. When she takes her mismatched shoes off to step into the slacks, I grab the matching shoe and throw the other one into her closet—no arguing. I brush her hair and gently wipe away the red from her eyebrows. I guess it was a lipstick pencil.

Thank God it wasn't a red marker.

"Y'all have fun! Tell Izzy and Jillian hi for me!" and off they go to Grandparents Day.

Mom loves Grandparents Day. She loves children. She loves her grandkids. I know this event will make her happy. I hope it lasts the rest of the day and through the weekend. But I know it won't. We only have short spurts of happiness. They fade away as fast as her memory.

"Tell Peggy about the little girl in Jillian's class," Dad says when they arrive home.

"Oh, Peggy, this beautiful little girl was sitting with the teacher all by herself. She looked so sad. I asked Jillian, "Where is her grandmother?" She told me she didn't come. I went over and gave her a big hug and invited her to sit with us."

"That was so sweet, Mom! You always have so much love to give!"

"What are y'all doing tonight, Dad?"

"We are meeting Erin and Scott at The Chimes, and y'all are welcome to join us for dinner."

"That sounds great. Let me check with Jimmy."

Soon, we are pulling out of the driveway and on our way to The Chimes. It's Erin's weekend to spend time with Mom and Dad. My three sisters each take a weekend, so every three weeks, they plan activities with Mom and Dad.

Well, mainly for Mom. They decided Jimmy and I need a break on weekends, and Dad needs a break on Saturdays during the day. They usually have dinner with them on Friday and Saturday evenings. On Saturday morning, they pick up Mom for mani/pedis, shopping, and running errands. Then, they have lunch or just take her to their house to hang out and get her to "help them cook," which isn't easy.

Jimmy and I don't have anything planned tonight, and dinner at the Chimes sounds fun. The restaurant is packed, and we have to wait 30 minutes to get a table. It is a casual local joint with great food, from burgers to seafood. We finally get seated and order dinner.

I looked at my cell phone and find a text from my friend Sera Bee, a fantastic bluesy piano player and singer. She is playing tonight at 8:00 p.m., down the street at a cool bar with a lovely courtyard.

"Jimmy, Sera Bee is playing tonight at Bottle and Tap!"

"Really? Let's go after dinner."

"Where are y'all going?" Scott, my brother-in-law, asks.

"To hear music. We should all go. It's down the street. Y'all will love Sera Bee, she is terrifically talented!"

"Dad, do you and Mom want to go hear some music? My friend, Sera Bee, is in town."

"That sounds good. Jimmy's driving, and I can have an after-dinner drink!"

My niece, Brennan, and her boyfriend, Mitch, are also with us and want to join. It's a party!

Sera Bee has driven over with her band from Mississippi. I met her at an event at the Sundance Film Festival in Park City a couple of years ago. She always lets me know whenever she plays in Baton Rouge or New Orleans. As we walk into the courtyard, Sera sees me and comes over to say hello. She is happy we came! She knows Mom has Alzheimer's and gives her a big hug.

We grab a great table right in front of the stage, and everyone orders drinks. Soon, the band begins playing, and Sera Bee blows everyone away. Erin and I grab Mom and dance in front of the stage. Scott is taking pictures, Jimmy smokes a cigar, and Dad sips his whiskey, smiling. He is grateful Mom is having fun. It's like old times. Mom has found her zest for life tonight. It's invigorating. It makes my heart sing.

"Peggy, this one's for your parents!" Sera Bee says from the stage and starts singing the Willie Nelson song, "You Are Always on My Mind."

"Dad, dance with Mom!" I called out.

He stands up and grabs her hand, and they walk to the front of the stage and begin slow dancing. Soon, they are swaying with their eyes closed. He is over 6 feet, and Mom is about 4'11", so he rests his chin on her forehead. Tenderhearted, loving, and dancing under the moonlight. It is a magical moment. Erin and I look at each other and start crying. I stand up, take a video and pictures with my iPhone.

"Enough with the pictures. Dance with me," Jimmy says, and we dance next to my parents.

My mother has always loved to sing and dance. None of the Sweeney sisters are shy about dancing. We have taken over many dance floors in our lives! We learned it from her. I feel free and lighthearted when I dance, and my spirit soars. My mom feels the same way, too.

Later that night, I watched the video of my parents dancing, then texted it to my sisters and my good friend, Carmen, in Los Angeles. They text back:

Aww, so wonderful!

Lovebirds!

Too sweet!

The next day, I texted my sisters:

Let's plan outings for Mom and Dad with music. I think it is healing for Mom. Let's find restaurants with music every week.

We scramble to find restaurants with music, and soon, every Friday, they are going to a restaurant with a band. Shannan gets tickets for musicals at Baton Rouge Theatre, and Kelly brings them to the symphony and the ballet. On each occasion, Mom is happy. Mom is our Mom again, at least for the night. I wish we could bottle the magic of music and pour it into her coffee. These are the moments we will cherish. These moments outweigh the bad ones.

Weeks later, Carmen mailed me a surprise: the photo of Mom and Dad dancing framed in a white wooden heart frame decorated in pearls. It is beautiful and touching. When I look at the picture, I hear Sera Bee singing and see my parents dancing cheek-to-cheek—so alive, so in love. They seemed so happy. Their eyes closed, remembering the good times. Their hands entwined, holding onto the love that will live forever.

These are the moments we cling to. They outweigh the bad ones. For a song, a dance, a fleeting night, my Mama is still here.

CHAPTER EIGHT
A BASKET OF MEMORIES

Mom, look what I found upstairs in the attic," I call as I come down the stairs, balancing various boxes labeled *Easter Decorations*.

"I forgot about those," Mom says.

I set the boxes on the table and head back upstairs for more. I was on a mission—excited to create a "good day" with her.

Mom sits at the table while I open the boxes and pull out bunnies, beautiful eggs, and other cute handmade treasures collected over the years. I remember her after-Easter raids at the Hallmark Shop returning with her prized loot. Mom was always hunting for a good deal! Now we "ooh" and "ahh" together, remembering past Easters. She's smiling, eyes bright. I feel as if we are unearthing a long-lost treasure chest.

"I remember when we made these for Stitches and Stuff," she says, holding delicate eggs they had blown out, dyed, decorated with pearls and other colorful jewels, then strung with pretty satin ribbons. The years have faded the colors—just like our memories.

Stitches and Stuff was her crafty circle of friends in the '70s. They'd gather in our back playroom to make holiday items sold at school fairs. When I was in college, I would drive across town from my sorority house to wash clothes and eat home-cooked leftovers, and I'd find the animated women crafting, gossiping, and laughing.

Their friendship has lasted more than 50 years. They still meet monthly for lunch at a local restaurant with their spouses. These women have watched my mom's slow decline.

"She seems just fine," they tell me. The denial is as thick as their love for her. Over the months, they began to accept it as she changed before their eyes. The slow progression is heartbreaking. Their beautiful, lively friend has become quiet and confused. They've witnessed firsthand how she argues with Dad at lunch and his frustration with her.

Recently, Miss Pat, one of Mom's closest friends, picked her up for lunch. Afterward, they got lost and drove around our neighborhood for an hour. Mom didn't remember how to get back to our house. Miss Pat called Dad to get the address. They laughed it off, but Miss Pat was stunned at how quickly Mom's memory was slipping.

I'm not sure when my parents last decorated for Easter. The Easter decorations fell away over time. We didn't notice when it happened. Like Mom's memory—at first, you don't see it. Then one day, it's undeniable. Poof! A gone pecan, as they say in Louisiana.

Well, this Easter will be different. The Easter fairy is in the house, determined to bring on the Easter parade. I feel my heart expand, and tears come to my eyes as I realize it doesn't take much to make Mom happy, at least for today. Her happiness breeds mine, and I welcome every speck of possible joy as the days stretch longer and are more challenging in the A-Zone.

Growing up in Baton Rouge, Easter was almost as big as Christmas in our family. We would scour the racks of Maison Blanche and D.H. Holmes for the perfect Easter outfits—dresses in pretty pastel colors with shiny patent leather shoes, white stockings, little white purses, gloves, and Easter bonnets with satin ribbons.

Our girls-only shopping extravaganza would include lunch at the Piccadilly Cafeteria. Moving down the line and choosing our Kids' Plate—an entree, two sides, a dessert, plus a hot, yummy yeast roll felt like heaven. All those steaming bins with the lovely ladies in uniform dishing food onto the sectioned China plates—it was fun and a little overwhelming.

"What are y'all having today, dawlin'?" they'd chirp, keeping the line moving.

"Aren't y'all pretty!"

"Let me guess, sweetie, you're the big sister, right?"

The four little Sweeney sisters dressed in beautiful hand-smocked matching dresses made by our Mama were a sight!

There was something special about deciding which colored Jell-O with fruit and whipped cream I would pick out for dessert. It was such a simple lunch, but I can still smell the delicious, chopped beef patty with gravy, the crispy fried chicken, the mashed potatoes swimming in butter, and the cooked-to-almost-mush green beans in bacon and onions. Southern cafeteria food, but somehow it felt like a feast! The thought makes my mouth water now. Let's make a trip to Piccadilly.

One of the servers would meet us at the end of the serving line, direct us to a table, and help my younger sisters with their trays.

I loved the piano player who would always smile at us while playing show tunes. My Mom would give us some change, and I would prance over and request something from *The Sound of Music* or *South Pacific*.

We couldn't wait to finish our lunch so we could slide our trays into the window with the automated conveyor belt to the dishwashers. Once, I stuck my head in the window and got bopped by someone's half-eaten spaghetti. My mom, sisters, servers, and the piano man howled while I stood mortified, trying to wipe my hair off with a napkin. I never did that again.

We never left Piccadilly without getting a chocolate green mint at the checkout stand. We thought they were free; years later, I realized my mother paid for them.

"Mama, look at these beautiful shoes! They'll go perfectly with my white eyelet Easter dress," I announced to the entire shoe department, holding bright yellow patent

136

leather shoes with a small, clear acrylic heel. They were magnificent, and at ten years old, I felt like Cinderella at the ball when I put them on my feet. I stood twirling around in front of a giant mirror with a young salesman nodding in approval.

"Peggy, I am not going to buy those. They are the tackiest shoes I have ever seen! What else would you even wear them with?" my mother said, and my 8-year-old sister Shannan stood by her side, nodding her head in agreement.

"I think they are cute!" six-year-old Erin chimed in. She always thought everything I wore or did was golden.

Mom tried to steer me to the simple white ballet flats—a step up from the juvenile Mary Jane shoes my little sisters were getting. I burst into tears and staged a drama-queen fit!

"If I can't have these, I don't want any! I'll wear my old scuffed-up shoes," I huffed, shoving the box away.

"Peggy, you are being ridiculous! Okay, if I buy them for you, you'd better wear them to church every week."

"I promise, Mama! Thank you," I said, floating out of the store with my "Cinderella slippers."

And I wore them until they pinched my toes. The joy of slipping those shoes on made me feel sophisticated and beautiful.

The last box contains the Easter tree Mom created when I was in high school—bare tree branches sprayed white. A few are bent, and the paint flakes, but I lift it out with reverence.

We both said, "Aww," at once and giggled. Mom rearranged branches and placed the tree in the center of the formal dining table. We hang faded pastel Easter eggs and admire our work. The only thing missing was our baskets.

On Good Friday, Mom used to boil dozens of eggs in a big pot with a white kitchen towel to keep the eggs from cracking. My sisters and I would gather around the kitchen table with coffee cups of colored-dyed water and use crayons to draw bunnies and flowers, writing our names before we dipped the eggs with the copper wire egg dipper. The large white wicker baskets with fake green grass would soon be filled with bright eggs. Miraculously, the ones with our names would appear in our baskets on Easter morning, and the rest would be hidden around the house when we woke up to see what the Easter Bunny had delivered!

Mom made the most beautiful Easter baskets I have ever seen. Around the large white or milk-chocolate bunnies in the middle, she tucked Elmer's Heavenly Hash, Pecan or Gold Brick Eggs, speckled robin eggs, bubble-gum eggs, and my favorite, the sugar diorama egg decorated with beautiful pastel frosting! She wrapped each basket with iridescent cellophane and topped it with a bright bow. Besides it sat a wrapped gift—a spring nightgown, pajamas, or stuffed bunny when we were younger. I always felt sorry for friends whose baskets weren't as grand as ours!

Mom follows me around the house as we decorate the living room with bunnies and eggs. We adorn the living room bookshelves, coffee table, side tables, and mantle. In the kitchen, we set up a crystal bowl with marble eggs on the table. Our holiday mentality was always "more is more."

"What are y'all doing down here?" Dad calls, coming down the stairs from his office.

"We are decorating for Easter!" Mom beams.

"It looks great," he smiles.

We're giddy. In another box, we find some pink, yellow, and baby blue netting—perfect for draping the chandelier. We hung more eggs. It's magical. We stand and look at our handiwork with awe.

I snap photos and text my sisters:

We are decorating for Easter! Y'all need to come to see it!

How cute! Erin texts.

We need to make plans for Easter Sunday. Mass at the Cathedral? Shannan texts.

Yes—let's keep it simple. Brunch at the Hilton after Mass! I'll make a reservation. Kelly texts.

Throughout the week, my sisters stop by to see our Easter parade of decorations.

"Come see what we did," Mom proudly exclaims, touring them through the rooms. Everyone admits they haven't decorated in years. When did life get so busy that we forgot to decorate for Easter?

Jimmy overhears and teases them. "How difficult would it be to put up your Easter tree? When I met y'all, every one of you had one," he says in his annoyed New Yorker tone. They laugh. They've learned to expect Jimmy's smart-ass comments.

I hate to admit it—I no longer have my Easter tree. When we moved back to Louisiana, I gave all our Easter decor to my friend, Christine, and her daughter, Makena. I wonder if they ever used it.

On Good Friday, Mom and I shopped our closets for Easter outfits since we are no longer shopping for new clothes. Outings with her have become too complicated, and we have plenty to choose from. I picked out a blue and white floral dress I bought in California a few years ago, and Mom chose a black dress. I'm horrified, as black is not "spring-appropriate" for Easter in Louisiana! I show her other options, but she is adamant about wearing the black dress. I finally convinced her to wear her pretty pink jacket on top. We will be styling in our pretty Easter outfits. The only thing missing is our Easter bonnets.

I wake up early on Easter morning. Getting ready has become challenging. I shower, do my hair and makeup, then go downstairs to help Mom with hers. She'd let me help her shower last night without arguing, and now she lets me primp her. She seems excited and looks beautiful.

"Look how pretty you look, Mom!"

"Where are we going?"

"It's Easter, Mom. We are going to Mass and brunch with the girls and their families."

"Oh, that's right. I forgot. Who's going to be there?"

"The whole family!"

"Really? Is Dad coming?"

"Yes, and Jimmy too."

"Where are we going?"

It doesn't end. Over and over, she asks the same thing, and I answer the same. It feels like *Groundhog Day*. It's maddening.

Then she sits in the living room across from Dad and tells him it is time to leave—ten times. I hear him tell her it's too early; Mass doesn't start until 11:30. She gets angry and storms away to her bedroom, slamming the door.

I'm setting Easter treats on the dining room table when I hear the commotion. I knock and let myself in. Thankfully, she hasn't locked it. She is lying in bed, staring at the wall. It breaks my heart to see her this way.

"Mom, the Easter bunny came! Come see."

She barely smiles but follows me out. Dad and Jimmy join us at the table where I have placed Easter cards and a "family basket" of candy. We open our cards and kiss each other Happy Easter! Dad immediately unwraps his favorite chocolate pecan Goldbrick egg and pops it in his mouth.

"These are much smaller than I remember," he says.

I grab a few bubble-gum eggs for the road. We head for the Cathedral downtown. Mom carries her old black purse with several candy eggs tucked into the top.

After all the decorating, the morning seems anticlimactic. I'm grateful we are meeting my sisters; we need a shot of Easter adrenaline. Unfortunately, the bubble-gum sugar isn't cutting it. In the back seat, I buckle Mom in. I watch as she unwraps a Heavenly Hash chocolate marshmallow egg, takes a small bite, and tucks it back into her purse. She leans her head back and closes her eyes.

By the time we arrive, my sisters have saved a long pew for us. We filed in, and everyone leaned in to kiss Mom and Dad. I sit beside Mom, and we sing with the choir. I hold the hymnal and trace the lines with my finger, but she doesn't need prompting. She remembers all the songs from attending Catholic schools. It amazes me. She can't remember what day it is or what we are doing today—but she can sing every word.

The music and being surrounded by her family lifted her spirits. Dad holds her hand, and I see her smile at him tenderly. She forgot she was mad at him less than an hour ago. Watching them interact this way reminds me that love survives through the madness of Alzheimer's. I turn and grab Jimmy's hand. He squeezes it, and I lean over to kiss him.

"I love you, Peggy Bug," he says.

"I love you too. Happy Easter, Jimmy Dean!"

We filed out of the church for the requisite family pictures before driving to the Hilton. Brunch is on the top floor overlooking the Mississippi River. A jazz band plays. The Easter bunny takes photos with the kids. My young nieces, Isabel and Jillian, and my nephew, Duncan, are mortified, but their mother—my sister Kelly—insists. Jimmy and I are laughing.

"That bunny creeps me out!" Isabel whispers, and we giggle.

I skipped the omelet station and head to the seafood station, piling my appetizer plate with shrimp, crab claws, and raw oysters. Kelly guides Mom to the Bloody Mary and mimosa station. I see her arguing with Mom, so I swoop over to see if I can help. Mom is confused about all the options. She grabs a slice of bacon with her hands and starts eating it.

"Mom, these are for the Bloody Mary's," Kelly says.

"I don't like Bloody Mary's. I like the other one!"

"I know—I'm getting you a mimosa," Kelly says, rolling her eyes at me as I grab a Virgin Mary. I plop a spiced green bean and okra into my glass.

"Thank you!" I whisper to her.

The buffet is lovely—so much easier than cooking, but I miss the family Easter dinners: bone-in ham cooked with Coca-Cola, pineapple rings, and mustard with brown sugar. And, the delicious sides of macaroni and cheese, layered salad, cheese grits, and squash casserole. Dessert was always a bunny cake with coconut icing perched on coconut-dyed green grass dotted with jellybean eggs. We loved helping Mama decorate the cake on top of an upside-down cookie sheet covered with aluminum foil. On the back patio, we would take turns at the old-fashioned ice cream churn, then crowd around with our mouths watering as Daddy lifted the top off, revealing vanilla ice cream dotted with fresh chunks of frozen peaches. Bunny cake topped with fresh peach ice cream is the definition of heaven. I want some now!

"Peggy, look at those beautiful hats," Mom whispers to me, eyeing the women at the next table.

"They're wearing their Easter bonnets, Mom!"

Before I can stop her, she's at their table telling them how beautiful they look. I jump up and follow. The two southern belles dressed to the nines are standing up at their table, having a lively conversation with my mother. They obviously enjoyed the unlimited mimosas.

"Would you like to try my hat?" one of the ladies asks.

"Sure," Mom says, and the lady settles her pink hat on her head.

"Why not?" I say when the other woman hands me her blue hat. I set it on my head. By chance, both Easter bonnets match our outfits—divine intervention. Now, all we need are white gloves. These Easter bonnets were the missing pieces of our Easter outfits. We smile at each other and stand a little taller with the colorful borrowed Easter bonnets on top of our heads.

My sisters stared, horrified. My teenage nieces are ready to crawl under the table.

"Kelly, take our picture," I say, and she hops up. Mom starts singing, "In your Easter Bonnet," and I chime in as we sashay around the table. The ladies sing along and want photos, too. We don't know all the words, so we make them up.

"Dad, come join us," and he stands reluctantly for a photo. Jimmy rolls his eyes and refuses to get up, so I walk over, throw my arms around his neck, and lean down. Kelly snaps away.

"Seriously? Can't I eat my lunch without a million Sweeney pictures?" he mutters under his breath as he flashes a practiced "Sweeney Smile" for the picture.

We reluctantly return the Easter bonnets to our new friends, who are now posing for their own pictures with Kelly as their photographer. Kelly agrees to email them some photos.

After demolishing the dessert bar—key lime pie, strawberry shortcake, pecan pie, and pretty pastel petit fours, the jazz band strolls over to our table, taking requests.

"Hello, Dolly?" I ask them. They launch into it while Mom and I jump up, holding hands, singing, and dancing together. We're having the time of our lives! The Easter Bunny comes over and joins us. My nieces bolt and run out to the lobby. My teenage niece, Peyton, scampers after them. Kelly keeps snapping.

Shortly after, the men gather at our table and divvy up the check. The room is being cleared out for the next brunch seating. Our Easter celebration winds down.

147

Outside at the valet, we bid each family farewell as they leave. Our car comes last, and Jimmy tips the valet while he opens the doors. Mom and I sit in the back; Dad takes the front. Jimmy is always our designated driver. We drove in silence back to the house across town. Mom leans her head back and closes her eyes. I took her hand and held it for the 20-minute drive.

Her hand is small and frail, blue veins raised beneath her skin. Behind my oversized sunglasses, I cry silently. I wonder if this will be our last Easter together.

Once home, we disperse—Mom to her room to lie down, Dad to his chair, Jimmy to the den to watch golf. I peel off my dress and pearls, pull on shorts and a T-shirt, and then slide under the covers. The emotional rumble rises; I press it down. It's easier to sleep.

Later that week, I mournfully pack up the Easter decorations while Mom is taking her afternoon nap. Jimmy helps carry the boxes up to the attic.

Mom never notices they're gone.

But new Easter memories—bonnets, mimosas, a jazz band, and a creepy Easter bunny—live in my mind as we celebrated one last beautiful Easter with my mother—all captured with Kelly's camera. In my heart, I place these

148

memories in a big Easter basket alongside my childhood memories, then I wrap the basket with iridescent cellophane, placing a big pink bow of gratitude on top!

Mom's Easter Baked Ham

Ingredients:

One fully cooked ham (8-10 pounds)
One large can of pineapple slices with juice
3 Tsp. of brown or Dijon mustard
3/4 cup of brown sugar
2 Tsp. of honey
One can of Coca-Cola

Instructions:

Heat oven to 325°F
Place the ham fat side up in a large roasting pan.
Score the ham with a sharp knife on the fat side and pour the Coke over it.
Decorate with ham, pineapple slices, and cherries, securing them with toothpicks.
Mix the brown mustard, honey, and brown sugar, then baste over the ham and fruit with a pastry brush.
Cover with foil, sealing around the edges of the roasting pan.
Place in the oven and cook for one hour and 30 minutes, occasionally basting with drippings.
Remove the foil from the ham, baste it with juices, and then place it back in the oven for 15 minutes.
Remove the ham from the oven and rest for 15 minutes before placing it on the platter and slicing.
Use pineapples and cherries as a garnish.

Yield

15-20 servings on a buffet, plus save the ham bone and make red beans

Family Notes:

We grew up having Mom's delicious, mouthwatering ham for Easter, but once Honey Baked Ham became popular, our family joined the bandwagon. Dad would order a Honey Baked Ham and a Honey Baked Turkey. Mom loved it because it was the easier, softer way, no clean-up, and the leftover ham was perfect for red beans and rice the following Monday. I recently went to a holiday party, and my friend Rawndy brought traditional Louisiana baked ham, but she used root beer. It reminded me of Mom's Coca-Cola ham. I need to make it for our next family party!

CHAPTER NINE
ROAD TRIPS TO NOWHERE

I'm standing in the kitchen making a salad for dinner when I hear my dad's van pull into the driveway. They're home from their trip to Memphis, Tennessee, and Rolla, Missouri. I open the back door, and Dad storms in—red-faced, furious, and visibly shaking.

"I've had it! I'm done," he says, heading straight for the bathroom.

Mom comes in behind him, obviously pissed off. I hugged her, still trying to figure out what's going on.

"Peggy, your father is crazy. I'm worried about him. He's been driving in circles for hours," she blurts, then storms to her bedroom, slamming the door.

"What happened?" I ask Dad when he comes out of the bathroom.

"Never again! She screamed at me for the last five hours that I was going the wrong way. 'You missed our stop,' she kept saying. I told her I'd call you to prove I knew the way home, but she grabbed my phone."

He pours whiskey on ice, takes a gulp, and collapses at the kitchen table. His breathing is shallow, his hands trembling. I have never seen my dad like this. Our protector, always in control, is crumbling right before my eyes. His blood pressure must be through the roof.

"I'm so sorry, Dad."

"I'm not sure if she threw my phone away when we stopped for gas, and she went to the bathroom."

"Let me check her purse."

Mom is in the bedroom, pulling clothes from her suitcase and tossing them onto the armchair.

"Mom, do you have Dad's cell phone?"

"No, I don't have it!" she says defiantly, as I dig through her purse and come up empty.

Jimmy arrives home and joins Dad in searching the car. They pull out the floor mats and toss them onto the driveway.

"Dad, do you have the Find My iPhone app?"

"I think Shannan set it up for me, but I'm not sure."

I called my sister. "Shannan, here's what's happening…"

"Let me try to find it on my laptop. I'll call you back."

Dad and Jimmy dig through the glove compartment and side door pockets. Dad is livid, his face flushed, his voice shaking.

"This is why you don't take an Alzheimer's patient on a road trip. Nothing good can come of it," Jimmy mutters, shaking his head.

The house phone rings. I see Shannan on the caller ID and grab it quickly, hoping Mom doesn't pick up. Too late—I heard her voice from the bedroom.

"Hello?"

"I'm on Find My Phone. It says the phone is in the house. It should be beeping," Shannan says.

"I didn't take his phone," Mom insists from the bedroom phone before slamming it down.

Jimmy heads back to the car, listening for the beep. Dad and I walk into the bedroom. Mom is lying in bed, casually reading *People* magazine. Suddenly, I heard a faint beep.

Dad and I look at each other with relief. I drop to my hands and knees, searching under the bed and dresser. Nothing. Dad checks the closet. The sound is muffled but close. I realize it's coming from her drawers. I open them one by one—jewelry, scarves, no luck. Then, in the second drawer, under a pile of underwear, I see it.

"Here it is, Dad!" I handed it to him. He exhales and shakes his head before turning to Mom.

"Sherry, you had it the whole time. How could you do something so mean? You hid my phone from me?"

"Dad, please stop," I warn, knowing this will only escalate.

"I didn't have your phone! I don't know how it got there! Stop blaming me for everything," Mom screams.

"It's OK, Mom. We found it, and that's all that matters."

Dad walks out with his phone. I follow.

I still have the house phone in my hand. Dad goes straight to his chair in the living room, downs the rest of his whiskey, and stares into space. A second later, I heard the bedroom door slam.

Shannan is still on the line. She's heard the entire exchange.

"We found it. I'll call you back."

"Please do," she says quietly.

Jimmy and I sit with Dad as he recounts the road trip from hell.

Over the last few months, Mom had begged Dad to visit her childhood friend Barbara in Missouri. My niece, Peyton, was in a summer internship at St. Jude in Memphis, so Dad planned the trip around both. They drove to Memphis on Thursday, had a lovely dinner with Peyton, and spent the night in a hotel. The next day, they continued to Rolla for the weekend with Barbara and her husband, Gary.

The visits were wonderful. Mom was thrilled to see Peyton and spend time with Barbara. But the drive home unraveled everything.

Dad had planned to stop in Memphis for sightseeing at Graceland and spend the night. But when they arrived, Mom was sound asleep, so he decided to keep driving straight to Baton Rouge. When she woke up just past Memphis, all hell broke loose.

"Where are you going? You missed our exit," she scolded.

She berated him for the next five hours, threatening to throw her Diet Coke at him, even threatening to jump out of the car. At one gas stop, she pointed at a police officer and said she'd tell him Dad was kidnapping her.

Dad warned, "If you do that, they'll put you in the hospital for observation for days."

By the time he made it home, he was shaken to his core.

"I'm so sorry, Dad. I should've gone with you," I whisper.

Later, I call Shannan and fill her in.

"She's putting them—and everyone else on the road —in danger. It may be time to think about Memory Care," she says, always the voice of reason.

"I know. I'm worried about Dad. I've never seen him like this."

When I tell Dad what Shannan suggested, he shakes his head. He understands, but he's not ready for such a decision.

I check on Mom. Her bedroom door is locked. I reach for the key above the door jamb and let myself in. She's sitting on the bed, pulling at the comforter.

"Mom, are you hungry? I made a big green salad, and we have chicken salad too."

"OK, I'm coming."

She joins me in the kitchen, and I hand her napkins and silverware. It takes her five minutes to set the table. The forks and knives land in a crazy pattern, but does it matter? Dad won't eat. Jimmy and I sit with her, and I ask about her visit with Aunt Barbara.

"Who?" she asks.

"Aunt Barbara and Gary—did you have fun at their house in Missouri?"

"We didn't see them."

"Yes, Mom, you went to see Peyton and Aunt Barbara."

"We saw Peyton. She was so happy! She loves working there."

158

I let it go. Later, I tell Dad she doesn't remember seeing Barbara. His shoulders sag.

"That's ridiculous. I'll show her the pictures tomorrow."

The next day, I find them sitting together on the old green sofa. He's scrolling through photos on his phone, showing her proof.

"That was years ago," she says flatly.

"No, that was this past weekend. You just don't remember."

"No, you don't remember! Why are you doing this to me?" she shrieks, storming out.

Dad and I exchange a weary glance. Neither of us speaks.

Life in the A-Zone is cruel. My strong dad is depleted, his health at risk. When will we learn not to argue or reason with her? In this world, reason is a lost cause.

Later, I found Mom crying in her bedroom.

"Mom, are you OK?"

"I just want to die," she cries out.

"Oh, Mom, please don't say that."

We stood hugging and crying together. I don't know what to say or what to do. I understand. Part of me wants to die, too. This is too frickin hard. We can't do this. We don't want to do this. I don't want to do this!

Days and weeks pass, and I forget about the trip from hell.

When my friend Kathryn offered me her theatre tickets to see the Broadway musical *Waitress* at the Saenger Theatre in New Orleans the following Sunday, I jumped at the opportunity. I am starving for live theatre—my favorite thing to do—and it's been way too long. Mom also loves theatre. We both love musicals. I've heard great things about *Waitress*, so I wanted to bring her for a wonderful mother-daughter day trip to New Orleans. I can't wait to tell her and go into planning mode.

We can have brunch before going to see the play. New Orleans offers so many great brunch options! I am looking for a restaurant near the theatre.

"Mom, do you want to drive to New Orleans to see *Waitress*, the musical at the Saenger? Kathryn gave me her tickets," I asked her at dinner that night.

"Yes, that sounds fun," she says.

160

"That was sweet of Kathryn. Your mother will love going to see the play. Where will you park?" Dad asks.

"I think we should park at the Ritz-Carlton, have brunch in their restaurant, then walk to the theatre. It's only two blocks away."

"That sounds like a great plan. I will give you some money for brunch and parking. Thank you for asking your mother. It will be a treat for her!" Dad says. I know he is grateful for a day to himself.

"It will be a treat for me too, Dad!" I replied. I mean it. I believe it. I want a beautiful mother-daughter day with my mom.

***

In 1987, I moved to New York City with $1,500 and big dreams of making it as an actress. I had recently been divorced and was living in Houston, where I worked in commercials, training films, commercial print work, and theatre, plus worked as a temporary secretary to supplement my bills.

My mother was the first to visit me in the one-bedroom sublet apartment in Chelsea. I worked as a temp in various law firms, barely scraping by on enough money for rent, food, acting class, and subway fare. I was lucky then to have seen one Off-Broadway play as a guest of an LSU theatre buddy who worked as the artistic director.

My mother scheduled her trip just five weeks after I had moved. I think she wanted to check on me. I wouldn't admit it, but I was lonely, and life in New York wasn't as glamorous as I had imagined. With Mom there, I knew I would finally be able to enjoy New York because she would spoil me. I planned our fun itinerary and didn't accept any work that week. I would play with my mom in my new city, even if I had to eat scrambled eggs and peanut butter sandwiches for a week after she left.

Mom and I went to see three Broadway plays, including *Dreamgirls* and the newly opened *Steel Magnolias* play, where we laughed and cried, and then, by chance, met the Louisiana playwright Robert Harling in the lobby!

We dined at the famous theatre restaurant, Sardi's, and I got an actor's discount with my Screen Actors Guild card. We walked down 5th Avenue window-shopping, sat people-watching on a park bench eating bagels in Washington Square, got lost in the Village, and ate at Carmella's, an excellent little Italian restaurant. They didn't serve alcohol at the restaurant, and we didn't know to pick up a bottle of wine beforehand, but my mom, who had never met a stranger, started talking to the young couple sitting next to us. Within minutes, they were sharing their wine with us.

After our fabulous Italian dinner, we went to a piano bar where Broadway actors sang show tunes. It was glamorous and intoxicating.

We ate New York hot dogs on the steps of the Metropolitan Museum before spending hours wandering the museum halls, where we fell in love with the Impressionists, especially the Degas Ballerinas. On Sunday morning, we attended Mass at St. Patrick's Cathedral, then took a cab to Tavern on the Green for a delicious brunch in the beautiful Crystal Room, filled with chandeliers in different colors, before going to a matinee of the ballet at Lincoln Center. We strolled through Central Park and stopped for a drink at the Plaza Hotel Oak Room bar.

It was a magical mother-daughter week. It was the New York I dreamed of, and I wasn't pinching pennies—I was living the life, and Mom treated me like a princess. The day she left, we went out for breakfast at a diner on the corner, then she insisted on taking me to the Gristede's grocery store to stock my refrigerator. We stood hugging outside my building, waiting for the car service to take her to LaGuardia Airport. As the car pulled up, we reluctantly separated, and she handed me an envelope with her leftover subway tokens and cash.

"You take this, Peggy. You need this more than I."

I watched her drive away, waving at me from the back window. Once back in my apartment, I felt empty and melancholy. I sat on the sofa and thought, why am I here? This city is overwhelming me. I felt paralyzed by my fear. But my dreams were bigger. I kept moving forward.

I think of those days in New York as I drove the 80 miles to New Orleans, listening to the '50s station on Sirius XM Radio. Mom is no longer singing along to the songs. She isn't talking to me. She isn't telling her stories anymore. I try to speak to her, and she barely replies. I remember how annoyed we would get when she told us the same stories over and over again just a few years ago. What were we thinking? I would give anything for one of her stories right now. The silence is suffocating and uncomfortable. I try to think of things to say to her, but my mind goes blank. She just stares out the window. This is going to be a long day.

"Peggy, how much longer?"

"About thirty more minutes, Mom."

"Where are we going?"

"To see the Broadway play *Waitress*. It is going to be wonderful, Mom."

"Where's Dad?"

"He's at home. We will see him after the play."

"What play?"

We pulled into the garage at the Ritz-Carlton to valet park the car. The restaurant is beautiful. The hostess shows us to our table, and Mom looks around the room.

"This is pretty," she says.

"Do you want a mimosa, Mom?"

"Sure."

"Do you want to split French toast and an omelet?"

"Okay."

I make small talk. Our food comes, and we eat in silence. The excitement of the day is gone. Maybe this wasn't such a good idea. I look at my watch. The play isn't for another hour. Damn.

I asked our waitress to take our photo. We smile our Sweeney smiles, but there's nothing behind them today. No joy. No happiness. We are sitting in this beautiful restaurant, enjoying a delicious meal, but I'm barely tasting the food and not enjoying the company.

I pulled out my phone, texted Dad, and sent him the photo.

We are having brunch. All is good. I lied in the text.

Have fun! He texts back.

Yes, sir. A barrel of laughter. A ton of fun.

By the time I pay the bill and stop at the bathroom, it's time to walk down the street to the Saenger Theatre. I see long lines of theatregoers waiting outside, slowly making their way through the doors.

"What are we doing here?" Mom asks.

"Going to see a play, Mom. It is going to be great!"

"Your tickets are up the stairs to the right in the upper balcony," the usher tells me.

"Is there an elevator?" I ask. I haven't been here since I was a kid.

"No elevators working. Sorry."

Mom and I make our way up a long flight of stairs. She isn't happy and is seriously pissed off once I tell her we have one more flight of stairs to go. We find our seats. We watch the crowds settle and stare at the stage while the orchestra warms up.

"Look at the set, Mom. It's a diner."

"That's cute." She looks through the program but doesn't read it. I don't think she can read anymore. My mother loved to read, and I think she owns every Danielle Steel book ever published. These days, she flips through magazines and barely looks at the newspaper. She used to work on crossword puzzles every morning. Those days are over. Scratch reading and crossword puzzles off her list. Her list gets smaller and smaller in the A-Zone.

What am I thinking? Her lists aren't getting smaller. There are no lists. She no longer has things to do. She no longer wants to do anything.

I remember the "to-do" lists she made on a yellow legal pad with recipes, shopping lists, people to call, and letters to write. I find those yellow pads around the house now—memories of what used to be. I also found notes to family and friends she wrote on a yellow page, possibly before writing them in a birthday card. Was she afraid of ruining the birthday cards? Did she know she was having problems writing? I also found cards she wrote and never sent. More clues that her Alzheimer's had set in long before we acknowledged it.

I have never been so grateful for a Broadway show to begin. Sing, please, sing. Dance, please, dance. I'm waiting for the magic of theatre to transform me and take me away from my reality for a few hours. It doesn't happen. She's bored and restless. She keeps sighing and staring at me. I pretend to enjoy the play. I want to enjoy the play. It's great. The songs are brilliant, with clever lyrics and touching ballads by the talented singer-songwriter Sara Bareilles. The script is engaging, but I'm not transformed. I'm not taken away. Sadly, my Broadway fix no longer works in the A-Zone. My expectations are slammed down by the uninvited third-party hovering over us like a black cloud in this majestic, historical theatre.

"Is it almost over?" she says loudly.

"Shhhhh," I tell her, shaking my head. The couple sitting in front of us turns and gives us a dirty look.

This is painful. This is not fun. This is not magical. This sucks.

At intermission, I need to go to the bathroom, and she thinks we are leaving, and the play is over.

"No, Mom. It's just an intermission," I tell her. I am determined to see the rest of the show.

We walk down the long flight of stairs and find the bathroom. For the first time in my life, I'm grateful for a long line to the toilet. It will fill the time. She is now pissed off at me that we aren't leaving. I feel cruel. We make our way back to our seats. She is glaring at me when the second act begins. She stands up after fifteen minutes.

"I'm leaving," she says.

"Okay, Mom, let's go." My resolve to see the entire show has collapsed. I wish I could transport us directly home on a magic carpet.

Never again. What was I thinking? I am an idiot. What did I expect?

Seriously, you thought you could take your mother with Alzheimer's to the theatre. Do you believe you can have a lovely mother-daughter day? Are you out of your mind? Yes, I'm out of my mind. I'm losing it big time. I'm frickin' nuts. I'm Cuckoo for Cocoa Puffs, as Jimmy would say.

We finally get our car from the valet and pulled out of the parking garage to head home. Please, Mom, take a nap,

I pray. But no—the trip from hell has begun. The unending questions:

"Where are you going, Peggy?"

"We are going home."

"You are going the wrong way?"

"No, Mom, this is the right way."

"Get off here!" she tells me, over and over again.

Her anxiety rises by the moment. I'm scared she will jump out of the car.

"Mom, we are going home to Baton Rouge. We are almost there. This is LaPlace. This is Sorrento. This is Gonzales. This is Prairieville," I say in a calm voice when all I want to do is scream.

And finally, "Here's the Highland Road exit, Mom. We will be home in ten minutes."

"How was the play?" Dad asks as we walk into the house. I just shake my head. Mom, furious with me, goes straight to her room and closes the door.

"How was the play?" Jimmy asks, coming into the kitchen.

I take the *Waitress* program out of my purse and toss it dramatically into the garbage can.

"It sucked. Never again." I turned and walked upstairs, holding back tears. I change out of my "mother-daughter day dress" and throw on some "I don't give a crap" sweats.

"Are you okay?" Jimmy asks tenderly, walking into the bedroom.

I can't even reply. The lump in my throat is strangling me. I just look at him and start to sob.

He hugs me and lets me cry.

"Breathe, just breathe," he says, holding me tighter as my body shakes.

"I don't think I can breathe anymore."

"Let's go for a walk." He takes my hand and leads me down the stairs, out of the house, down the path to my beautiful lake—my serenity spot.

We walked out to the lake, sat on the park bench, and I told him about the day.

"All I wanted was a wonderful day with my mother. Is that too much to ask? Is that even possible anymore?" I plead. I want him to give me the answers.

"I don't know, Peg. I don't know."

"I no longer recognize my mother, and I no longer recognize me."

We sit watching the sun go down and then walk back to the house in silence. I find my mother and father in the living room watching TV.

"Where have you been all day?" Mom asks me.

I realize she doesn't remember we went to New Orleans, doesn't remember brunch, and doesn't remember the play. She doesn't even remember she was mad at me. The beautiful mother-daughter day I had planned for us doesn't exist in her mind.

It's hard enough to handle a regular day, but now I realize it's also challenging to handle special days. There will be no more special days. That part of our relationship has died. It's now just life maintenance in the A-Zone. We are in survival mode—a day at a time, an hour at a time, sometimes a minute at a time.

Like my parents' trip to Missouri, our mother-daughter trip to New Orleans was a trip to nowhere. Mom has forgotten, and Dad and I are left with emotional hangovers of disappointment and despair. Sadness weighs on our hearts like boulders of grief.

We continue to stumble, and we fall. It forces us to face our weaknesses and dig deep for the courage to keep moving forward. Will we run out of courage, or is it an unlimited supply? Will spirit refill my courage well? Is that what grace is? Alzheimer's—the great awakening—has brought us to our knees, and the only thing left to do is pray.

Dad and I are grasping at straws that crumble into a million little pieces in our hands—leaving us with nothing but the dull pain of emptiness. How many more straws will we continue to grasp?

How many more times will we take a trip to nowhere?

CHAPTER TEN
THE BIRTHDAY CRUISE

Our family has two July birthday queens—my baby sister, Kelly, and me. She was born on July 20th, and I was born on July 21st, eight years and one day apart.

When the obstetrician told Mom her due date was July 21, she said, "Oh no, having this baby on July 21st will not work. Peggy would never want to share her birthday."

He must have thought she was nuts. But he complied, and Kelly was induced on July 20th. My mother did everything she could to make our special days extra special, and I'm sure planning two birthdays back-to-back was difficult! But as adults, we cherish celebrating together and have made birthday memories in all the cities I've lived in— Houston, New Orleans, New York, Los Angeles, and now back in Baton Rouge.

174

Tonight, Kelly and I sit beside each other, surrounded by Mom, my sisters, our nieces, and our girlfriends as they sing Happy Birthday to us. We blow out the candles together on our beautiful petit four cake, then pose cheek to cheek for a picture before taking more photos with Mom and the entire group. We love pictures!

Kelly hands me a gift bag, and I'm shocked when I pull out tickets for the upcoming Taylor Swift concert in New Orleans, along with her latest CD. The tickets are right in front of the stage. I will join Kelly and her two young daughters, my nieces Isabel and Jillian. Kelly always spoils me.

Shannan organized this lovely birthday dinner at Erin's house, followed by a movie night to see *Mamma Mia 2!*

At the movie theater, we take up an entire row, passing large buckets of their addictive popcorn down the line. I pull Dollar Tree candy from my handbag and pass along Raisinets, Starburst, and Swedish Fish.

The movie is fabulous and perfect for a Girls' Night Out. Mom loves all our friends, and they dote on her. She sings along, claps, and is thrilled the entire night.

My friend Lea Ann elbows me, whispering, "I can't believe your mom knows every song!"

"I know, unbelievable, right?"

"That was so much fun. My birthday is next week," Mom says as we drive home.

"No, Mom, your birthday is in October. It's a few months away."

"No, it's next week," she tells me.

"Okay, Mom, we can plan something fun!"

It takes me a while to play the Alzheimer's game. Over and over again, I forget. One minute she is like my old mom, and within minutes we are back in the A-Zone. I can't help myself. I'm constantly trying to correct her and then realize—what is the difference?

For the past six months, every time someone has a birthday, my mother announces, "It's my birthday too!"

"When's my birthday party?" she asked me.

"Now I know where you get your birthday obsession," Jimmy tells me. He is constantly amused and teases me about it.

"Peggy doesn't have a birthday or a birth month, but a birth quarter," he tells my friends.

"You are an adult, Peggy! You don't need to celebrate all summer with different sets of friends and family," he tells me every year.

"And your point is?" I reply.

I'm wondering if Mom knows something we don't. Is this going to be her last birthday? Maybe we do need to celebrate earlier this year.

"Erin thinks we should take your mom on a cruise for her birthday weekend!" Dad tells me one night in September while I'm fixing dinner.

"A birthday cruise sounds fun, and Mom would love it!"

We have been on two Thanksgiving family cruises over the years, and we all agree it is the perfect Sweeney vacation.

"Y'all are human doings, not human beings," Jimmy tells me.

Everything and anything on the cruise itinerary appeals to us. On our first cruise, we didn't stop. From morning until late at night, it was go, go, go. We cruised out of New Orleans with fun Louisiana bands on board and a Catholic church group that brought along their parish priest.

Each morning, we met my parents at Mass at 7:30 a.m., followed by breakfast in the formal dining room. The days at sea were filled with endless activities, plus pool and spa time. At one point, Jimmy and I bailed out of the after-lunch bingo in the theatre with the family and went to our cabin to take a nap. We had just fallen asleep when my niece, Mackenzie, called us on the ship phone.

"Aunt Peggy, come meet us in the piano bar for Broadway trivia!"

"What time?"

"Now! We won't win without you!"

"Just because it's on the itinerary doesn't mean you have to do it!" Jimmy tells me when I left to join them.

"They need me."

We were very proud of our Broadway Trivia Trophy!

Jimmy bowed out of our second Thanksgiving family cruise seven years later and went to visit his parents. His father was in a nursing home with Alzheimer's, and he felt he needed to be there. Thank God, because his parents would be deceased by the next Thanksgiving.

"Do you and Jimmy want to join us for the birthday cruise? I would appreciate the help with your mom," Dad says as he watches me take the meatloaf and sweet potatoes out of the oven.

"We can't afford it right now, Dad. Plus, Jimmy is not a fan of cruises. He would rather go to a resort and play golf."

"Well, it's only four nights out of New Orleans, and if you come with us, you could stay in our room. I will treat you," Dad says, trying to convince me.

"That sounds great, Dad. Let me check with Jimmy."

"That's a good idea. A cruise with an Alzheimer's patient. Seriously?" Jimmy says, looking at me as if I'm insane. He sits and listens while I make my case that this may be the last chance to celebrate Mom's birthday.

"You see her declining. We need to make this birthday extra special. She will love all the shows and music."

"I understand. You should go, Peg. I'm sure your dad will appreciate it."

A few days later, Dad said he could upgrade to a suite if Jimmy wanted to join us. Later that night, I begged him to come with me.

"You can sit on the deck with Scott and smoke cigars while Erin and I go to the activities with Mom and Dad. We can go to the late-night adult comedy club and the piano bar after they are in bed. Please come, Jimmy. It will be fun and a chance to have a little vacation."

"Sure," he reluctantly agrees. He knows I'm struggling emotionally these days, and he probably would jump off the Mississippi Bridge if it would bring a smile to my face.

My other sisters, Shannan and Kelly, can't make the cruise. It will be just the six of us: my parents, Erin and her husband, Scott, Jimmy, and me.

We tell Mom, and she is thrilled. She forgets, and we tell her again—over and over. The day before we leave, I come home to find Mom and Dad's suitcases packed and, in the foyer, ready to go. I panicked because I was planning to help her pack. I'm certain her suitcase has all the wrong clothes. As she watches TV with Dad, I slip into their room, shut the door, and repack her suitcase. She probably won't even realize it. I step out of their bedroom just as she's about to go to bed.

Early the following day, we pick up Erin and Scott and drive to New Orleans. At the cruise port, Jimmy drops us off at the entrance with our suitcases and goes to park the car. Dad has upgraded us to VIP status, and we are sent directly to the front of the line, but then have to wait in the VIP lounge until we can board. While waiting, I see a photo-op with a ship backdrop and a cruise photographer taking pictures.

"Mom and Dad, come take a picture." I pull out my cell phone and snap a picture of them behind the photographer.

"No personal cameras are allowed here. You can order the photos at the Photo Salon on the lobby deck, the second floor," the photographer says.

Of course, we can, and, knowing my mom, she will purchase all of them for $25 a picture. But it was too late. I got the shot! I texted the photo to Shannan and Kelly.

Y'all have fun!

Wish we were going!

Jimmy arrives at the VIP lounge and grabs coffee and a donut.

"Come take a picture with me," I ask.

"No pictures. It's too early!" he snaps. He is already annoyed with the long lines trying to park in the garage, the wait to load onto the ship, and he's probably having a low-blood-sugar moment.

Forty-five minutes later, we are on the ship, taking another photo as we board and heading to our suite.

"Let's meet on the pool deck for lunch and drinks," Erin says, waiting for the elevator. They are staying one flight down.

We open the door to our suite to find over-the-top birthday balloons with streamers hanging from the ceiling, a chocolate birthday cake, and a birthday cruise gift bag. Dad wanted this to be an extra-special birthday for Mom and ordered the birthday package—the whole shebang.

"Happy Birthday, Mom!" I say as we step into the suite. She is thrilled.

"This must be the wrong room. We were supposed to have a suite!" Dad exclaims, glancing around at the "pretend suite." It looks like a standard room.

"Let me get the valet," I say, coming to the rescue, and walk out the door, avoiding eye contact with Jimmy. I found a valet two doors down and told him we were supposed to have a suite. He follows me to the room and confirms that this is a junior suite. It's one room with a sofa that, he tells us, will fold out. Jimmy sits on the couch, looking like his head is about to explode. He just shakes his head and rolls his eyes.

Dad stands there arguing with the valet about the suite and asks if we can move to a larger one or find another room for Jimmy and me.

Mom stands there, oblivious to what is going on, pulling the birthday streamers off the ceiling and throwing them on the bed and floor.

"Sorry, sir, the cruise is sold out. Let me know if there is anything else you need," the valet says as he scampers out of the room.

Where are y'all? Erin texts.

Problems with the room, I text her.

We are coming up to your room now, she texts.

We need another room—or about twelve more feet. When we pull out the sofa to make the bed, we will barely have enough space to walk between the beds to get to the bathroom. Luckily, the bathroom has a separate dressing area with an extra sink. There's a small balcony with two chairs facing each other, because there isn't enough space for them to face the ocean. These will be extremely tight quarters for four nights.

Mom is oblivious to the stress in the room. She looks at her birthday cake and digs through her gift bag. She pulls out a beach towel, a tumbler, and a box of chocolates. She holds up the beach towel.

"Look how cute! Let's cut the cake," she chirps. There is a childlike wonder to her energy—the complete opposite of the tension in the room.

"Later, Mom, we need lunch."

We hear the door knock. Jimmy jumps up to open it. Erin and Scott stand there, ready to see our "suite" and the birthday decorations.

"Happy Birthday, Mom!" they exclaim. I'm grateful for the distraction as I pull Jimmy into the bathroom.

"Come on, Jimmy, let's make the best of it. We probably won't be in the room much anyway, and when we come back at night, they will already be asleep," I assure him. He just looks at me.

"Is it Cigar O'clock?" Scott asks Jimmy, trying to break the tension as we walk out of the bathroom.

"Yes, it's Cigar O'clock!" Jimmy replies, pulling out two big cigars from his travel humidor, and we walk out the door.

Up on the pool deck, we smell burgers grilling, so we line up at Guy's Burger Joint to order burgers with steak fries, then stop at the condiment bar. Jimmy is now content, ready to enjoy a juicy bacon cheeseburger before his dessert cigar.

We find a table, and a waiter comes over to take our drink orders. Soon, Mom is sipping a piña colada with a pink umbrella. Dad enjoys cold beer. A calypso band plays next to the pool. Our juicy burgers are dripping with melted cheddar cheese, caramelized onions, and bacon grease. They are beyond delicious. Mom is happy. Dad is happy. Jimmy is happy. I'm happy!

We are good. All is well in our world. Maybe the cruise was a great idea.

"Hot, Hot, Hot," Jimmy says, nodding toward the calypso band, and we laugh. Nobody gets the joke, so we fill them in.

Years ago, we attended Jimmy's childhood friend Alec's wedding in Miami with Jimmy's sister, Kathy, and her husband, Pat. A calypso band by the hotel pool played the same songs repeatedly all day long for the entire weekend, including "Hot, Hot, Hot." Every time they played it, we laughed hysterically. We were ready to throw the band in the pool by the end of the wedding weekend.

Just as we finish our fabulous burgers, the calypso band starts playing "Hot, Hot, Hot," and we all roar with laughter.

"Are we having fun yet?" I say to Jimmy. He smiles. The ice is broken, and he is eager to get to the cigars on the top deck with my brother-in-law.

Back in the room, our luggage has been delivered, so we unpacked. I cut Mom and me a slice of chocolate birthday cake before going back upstairs to the pool. Jimmy never makes it back to the room to unpack. It's a two-cigar afternoon for him.

At 4:30 p.m., the ship pulls away from the dock in New Orleans, and we all stand on the top deck watching the French Quarter as we sail by. Jimmy stands behind me with his arms around my waist.

"There's our Cathedral," I say as we pass Jackson Square and the St. Louis Cathedral.

"Yeah, you're right!" he says. "Twenty-six years next month." We both remembered our wedding in the Cathedral. It seems like a lifetime ago. I want those days back. Living in New Orleans back then seemed so carefree.

"You owe me big time for coming on this cruise," he announces.

"You think?" I reply.

"Yes, I'm thinking of a week in Palm Springs for golf!"

"Good luck to you," I say, and we both laugh.

As the ship sails down the Mississippi River to the Gulf of Mexico, we head to the theatre to see the Welcome Show. It's a casual night, so we are all wearing the same clothes we had on this morning. I'm grateful I don't have to argue with Mom to change into something fancier.

The entertainment is fun, and Mom is in her element. She loves music. She smiles and claps, moving in her seat.

In the Grand Dining Room, the hostess seats us at our table by the window. Erin has brought a couple of bottles of excellent wine on the ship, so she, Scott, and Dad share a bottle of red. Mom has her mimosa. Jimmy and I split a large bottle of Pellegrino, and we ordered shrimp cocktails, Caesar salads, steaks, and hot chocolate lava cake with whipped cream. Mom orders shrimp fettuccine, and Dad orders a steak.

Everything is lovely until the entrées arrive, and Mom insists she ordered a steak, not the shrimp fettuccine. Dad argues with her until the waiter overhears and gladly offers to bring him another steak. Mom happily eats his steak. He eats her shrimp fettuccine until his second steak comes.

"It's a cruise, Dad. Chill. You can order as many appetizers or entrées as you like. This is her birthday. No need to fight with her," I whisper.

"Let her have it," Jimmy says under his breath.

"You're right! I need to chill," Dad says.

"Chillax," Scott says.

"Let's open the other bottle of wine," Erin says, changing the subject.

Mom and Dad want to return to the room after dinner. It has started to rain, and the boat is rocking. I'm feeling queasy, so we go to the infirmary and get some Dramamine, then meet Erin and Scott at the piano bar. They sing along, and I drink 7-UP, trying not to get sick.

We get back to the suite after midnight. Our sofa bed is pulled out, and we try to get undressed and ready for bed quietly, but Mom wakes up. She comes into the bathroom while I'm brushing my teeth. She needs to use the bathroom. She is confused—the flush button is on the back wall behind the toilet, not the usual handle on the side. When you flush, it makes a loud, obnoxious noise as the water is vacuumed down. She looks scared when I demonstrate how to flush it and then gets mad at me.

"I can do it. I'm not stupid," she says defiantly. I leave and close the door to give her privacy. She comes out after about ten minutes, and I see her put something under the bed. Note to self: check under their bed tomorrow.

Mom and Dad are up early and leave for breakfast. As soon as they shut the door, I jump out of bed and check under their bed. I found wadded-up toilet paper. I'm shocked. I retrieve it and place it in the garbage can. I take the plastic liner out and tie it up securely. I bring it out to the hall and find our valet.

"Can you please throw this away? My mom has Alzheimer's. Could you please give us extra liners and toilet paper? We would greatly appreciate it." He nods and smiles.

Now that is good service, I think, as I step back into the room. I moved the small garbage can to the side of the toilet instead of the dressing area. The reality hits me. I'm shaking. My mom doesn't know how to go to the bathroom anymore. I have read about this in the stages-of-Alzheimer's book. They lose all sense of toileting skills. I'm not sure what stage this is, but does it matter?

OMG! She couldn't remember how to flush the toilet. Maybe it scared her. I imagine her staring at the toilet while she tries to figure out how to flush. My poor mom. Was she embarrassed to ask me for help? Was she ashamed?

My heart goes out to her. This is so unfair. Alzheimer's, you suck!

I wake up Jimmy to tell him.

"Wow. I'm sorry. Come here," he says, pulling me back into the bed and holding me.

"This is why they tell you not to take Alzheimer's patients out of their homes. It's the disease, Peg, it's not your mom," he reminds me.

"I'm hungry. Let's go get some pancakes," I say. I need to eat my feelings, and a cruise is the perfect place to do it.

"And bacon. Lots of bacon and sausages," he says.

We head to the buffet dining room and pile our plates with eggs, pancakes, bacon, sausage, and fresh fruit. The waitress brings us juice and coffee. We don't see my parents in the dining room, but as we walk out to the pool deck, we see them lying in two lounge chairs holding hands. Their eyes are closed. I snap a picture.

"Aww. It looks like y'all love each other!" I tease, and they open their eyes and smile. Erin and Scott walk up in their bathing suits with cocktails in their hands. It's 10:00 a.m., and they are on vacation!

"Y'all go get your bathing suits on and join us," Erin says.

Soon, we are spread out on the deck with six lounge chairs, books, magazines, and drinks. It is a relaxing day and just what we need. Every time the calypso band plays "Hot, Hot, Hot," we laugh.

Mom lets me help her shower late that afternoon with no fight.

"I feel great!" she says as I put makeup on her and fix her hair. We get dressed up in colorful resort wear. For the last few months, I have had to fight with her every few days to take a shower. It's a nightmare. I'm grateful there is no fight tonight.

The theme of the evening show is "Around the World." We are going to the 7:30 p.m. show before Mom's birthday celebration dinner at 9:00. Dad, Mom, and I arrive early at the theatre and save seats in the first row. Jimmy, Scott, and Erin soon join us, and the cocktail waitress brings us frozen tropical drinks.

"This is your birthday show, Mom," I tell her.

"Really?"

"Yeah, Mom, we ordered it just for you!" Erin pipes in.

The cruise director, dressed in a colorful tuxedo, greets us, and we tell him it's Mom's birthday.

"We have a great show planned for you!" he says to Mom.

Mom is glowing! She loves the attention. We take pictures of her with the cruise director, and he takes a group picture of us. The show starts, and she is ecstatic. She claps and sings along for most of the numbers. The musical revue takes us on a journey around the world and ends with fireworks and streamers. The singing, dancing, and sets are excellent— "Broadway-worthy," I think.

"This was wonderful! How did y'all plan this?" she says.

Mom believes this show was just for her! The childlike wonder and sparkle in her eyes is the money shot for the entire cruise. She hugs the cruise director when she sees him at the door, and he wishes her happy birthday again. It is her night. The birthday dinner is excellent and ends with champagne and cake. The servers come over and sing Happy Birthday. Mom radiates joy and smiles. Dad is happy too, and for a few hours, we all forget about her Alzheimer's.

The next day, the cruise stops at Cozumel. Dad doesn't think they can make the long walk to a beachside resort we visited years before. The rest of us want to go to the resort, which offers a very reasonable price for a nice pool with snorkeling equipment, drinks, and lunch. We feel guilty leaving Dad with Mom on the ship, so we compromise and ask them to join us for margaritas, chips, and salsa at one of the Mexican restaurants in the tourist shopping area right down from the dock. Mom is tired and quiet that day. She seems off. I believe the cruise is starting to take its toll on her.

We exit the boat and find a restaurant. We sit on the outside patio overlooking the gorgeous ocean, and the waves crash onto the side of the deck. After a margarita, they are ready to return to the boat. They are tired and ready for a nap. We hug them goodbye and eagerly head to the resort.

"Let's party!" Scott says as we watch them walk away holding hands. We see Dad flag down a pedicab, and off they go.

I feel guilty for walking away, but we need an afternoon to relax and not worry about Mom.

"They will be fine," Erin says. "She looks tired, and they need to rest."

"I hope so."

We walk a mile down the road to the resort, pay the entrance fee, change into bathing suits, and walk out to the pool. We have about an hour in the sun before the weather changes fast, and it starts to pour. We ducked into the beachside hotel restaurant for a fajitas lunch. As soon as lunch is over, the rain stops; Scott and I jump into the ocean with our snorkeling gear. Jimmy enjoys his cigar. Erin has a massage at the spa. The water is way too rough to snorkel. Scott and I jump back in the pool. It's a carefree afternoon, and we are grateful for some chill time. The weather report is not good, and we make our way back to the ship just in time. Five minutes later, it begins to storm. I stumbled upon Mom and Dad in the main lobby bar listening to music and enjoying cocktails. They look animated and have made friends with another couple.

"How was Mom today?" I ask Dad.

"She was tired, so she slept most of the day."

"Well, she seems rested and happy, Dad. I'm glad y'all had a good day."

We meet later in the piano bar and find Mom singing along. And it is even better when we discover the show in the big theatre is a New Orleans theme tonight. Mom is in her element since these are the songs she grew up singing. They bring her back to her childhood. It's touching to see her so engaged.

After dinner, to our surprise, Mom and Dad announced they wanted to go to the Adult Comedy show with us.

Probably not a good idea. I think.

"This should be interesting," Jimmy whispers as we go to the comedy lounge and look for a table. It's crowded, and we have to sit at different tables. Dad and I sit with Mom and another couple at a booth right in front of the stage. Jimmy is across the room with Scott and Erin. The show begins with a raunchy comedian from New York. Mom and Dad are laughing hysterically, along with everyone else. However, my mom has an unusual laugh, and she can't stop laughing even when the crowd quiets down. The comedian starts to heckle her, and she howls more. Her laugh goes on and on. The entire audience is now laughing at Mom's laughter more than the comedian. I look over at Jimmy, Scott, and Erin across the room. They are hysterical.

The comedian ends his set, and the next comedian comes on. Mom is having a great time and doesn't want to leave, even though it is after midnight, so Dad orders another drink. The people we were sitting with left, and Erin, Scott, and Jimmy moved to our table. The second comedian is even raunchier. I want to crawl under the table at some of his jokes. Erin and I exchange glances, flinching. OMG!

"This is embarrassing," I whisper to her, and we laugh at how crazy it is to sit with Mom and Dad and listen to these dirty jokes. They don't seem embarrassed at all.

"That was great," Mom says as we leave. Jimmy approaches the comedian and begins discussing New York.

"The old country in my family was Brooklyn and Queens," I hear Jimmy tell the comedian.

Erin and Scott go to the casino, and Mom and Dad go to bed. Jimmy and I grab cappuccinos and gelato at the coffee bar, then walk to the pool deck. It's a beautiful night. The stars are shining, and there is a lovely salt-air breeze. An animated movie is playing on a massive screen over the pool. We find two lounge chairs away from the crowd, sip our cappuccinos, and eat our gelato.

"I haven't laughed that much since we moved back to Baton Rouge," I tell Jimmy. "Watching my mom and dad laughing together instead of arguing is a treat. Can we bottle this fun and take it home?"

"You will treasure these memories with your parents for the rest of your life. I think your mom enjoyed her birthday," Jimmy says.

"Do you think it is going to be her last birthday?" I ask him.

"I don't know, Peggy but if it is, just know that it was special."

"We made her laugh, sing, dance, and smile. Best birthday cruise ever!"

"And you have the pictures to prove it," he teases me.

"Thank you, Jimmy, for coming with me! It means the world to me."

"I'm happy I came."

I smile at him, and I know he means it. He takes my hand and pulls me over to his chair.

"Laissez les bon temps rouler, dahlin'," he says.

"Yeah, you're right, Cher—let the good times roll, Jimmy Dean," and we kiss under the stars.

CHAPTER ELEVEN
WALKING AWAY

Beep-beep, beep-beep is our new normal. We've now set the home security to beep twice whenever we walk in or out, serving as a constant reminder that Mom has the Big A. We set it to warn us she could be walking away from home. Walking away or running away is the big question!

I read about Alzheimer's patients walking out of their homes on an Alzheimer's Facebook support page, and it's no surprise that it is happening. However, once we set the alarm to the double beep, it confirmed that Mom was getting worse.

The light of day slips away. Our status quo snuck out in the dead of night, and we didn't notice it. Come back, please! I'm not ready for more change.

I searched the internet for the stages of Alzheimer's. I want to know what to expect and recognize the signs. I don't think my mom is following these steps. Are we on step 3 or step 5? What happened to step 4? Maybe we skipped a few steps and are on steps 6 or 7. It's like the Chutes and Ladders game we played as kids, and I don't want to play it. I'm standing with crossed arms, stomping my feet in defiance.

We have a good day, and we think maybe she isn't so bad, then the next day is awful, and we slide down the chute. Down we go and land abruptly on our butts. Ouch, that hurt! We shakily pull ourselves up by the bootstraps and carry on. We don't have a choice.

What's the alternative? Get in the car and drive away. Far away. Back to sunny California? I often think about the beaches, my neighborhood park, our brightly painted condo, our courtyard, our old comfy blue sofa, our pretty blue bedroom, and our friends.

I long for breakfast at our neighborhood diner, Nat's Early Bite, three blocks from our house. We would walk in, and they would call us by our names. Jimmy swears they are the best pancakes, golden brown and perfectly cooked. I crave their homemade turkey sausage egg scramble with spinach, mushrooms, and cheese, topped with their homemade salsa, along with their crispy home fries and toast with homemade apricot jam!

I miss Friday nights at La Fogata, our hole-in-the-wall neighborhood Mexican restaurant, where you ordered at the counter and then helped yourself to the salsa bar with the crisp pickled carrots and onions. Their Chile relleno was legendary, and I ordered it every time.

I think about Porto's Cuban Bakery. I crave their incredible iced tres leches coffee, the potato balls filled with deliciously seasoned ground meat, guava turnovers that melt in your mouth, buttery cinnamon coffee cake, and heavenly chiffon mango cake. We would drive out to Burbank on Saturday mornings, scramble for parking in the overcrowded lot or on the street, stand in long lines out the door trying to figure out what to order, and walk out with boxes of their delicious treats.

Sometimes we would have lunch at Porto's—delicious hot Cuban pressed sandwiches with crispy plantain chips—ordered at the counter, then join a line for a table. Afterward, we would get in the other bakery line for coffee and our boxes of pastries for dessert. It was pure indulgence, and there isn't anything like Porto's in Louisiana!

I recently heard they ship frozen potato balls and pastries. Sounds great, but it wouldn't be the same. The charm is going there to experience the noisy, happy vibe behind and in front of the counter.

Our lifetime of stuff is still in storage in California. We thought it would only be a month or so before we would call the movers for the delivery and move into our own place. Best-laid plans? Yeah, right. It's been two years with no call and no delivery. We have settled with my parents for the long haul. I can't abandon my father in the A-Zone.

Will we ever see our stuff again? I think about our artwork, my books, China, cookbooks, bedspread, and more. Everything I packed up, wrapped in bubble wrap, and slipped into a box seems trivial now. Some days, they pop into my brain out of nowhere. I tell myself it's just stuff. The monthly charges on our bank card keep adding up. By this time, we could have bought all brand-new stuff! If we haven't needed it for this long, maybe we never will.

It's just part of the insanity of life in the A-Zone. Living with a loved one with Alzheimer's forces you to live in the moment, but I want to live in the past, or dream of the future. I don't want to be in the here and now. It's too painful.

In the news, there are fires all around Los Angeles, including the San Fernando Valley, where our belongings are stored, and I wonder what would happen if the movers' storage facility were to burn down.

"It's time to get our stuff here! What if it burns in the L.A. fires?" I tell Jimmy in a paranoid panic.

"I know. We should," Jimmy mutters, but we do nothing.

We don't have the energy to deal with it. Not now. Not today. Maybe next week, next month, next year. We are treading water in an ocean of depression. Everything seems exhausting.

I wonder if I would feel relief or sadness if our stuff burned in a fire. I would feel a bit of both. When this is over, we can start fresh. Just sell everything and move on. What do we need to exist after our life in the A-Zone? Everything seems frivolous now. Our old life is so far away. Maybe I wouldn't like my stuff in my new world anyway.

Will I even like myself? Who will I be after our life in the A-Zone? Who will Jimmy be? Who will we be as a couple? Who will my dad be? Who will my sisters be? Who will our family be?

I try to understand Mom's motive for walking away from the house. She's bored, she's frustrated, she's angry, she's sad, she's irritable, she's restless, she's confused, she's just DONE! She picks up her purse and walks out. She tells Dad, after the fact, that she was going to see her mom, or Barbara, her friend in Missouri, her brother, who lived in Sweden and passed away last year, or various friends who live across town.

Maybe my mother just can't stand living with us anymore. Is it too hard to see herself drifting away, or is it too hard for her to watch our sad reactions to her slipping away?

"I hate you. You are the meanest man I've ever met. I want a divorce. I'm going to get an apartment with my mother," she says almost daily to my father as she storms off to her bedroom. He is so hurt. I can see it in his eyes.

"I'm so sorry, Dad. You know she loves you. Please forgive her. It's just the disease talking," I say, telling him the exact words Jimmy says when I'm upset with her nastiness.

"I know, you're right," Dad says, sighing deeply.

My mother walks out of the house with her black purse, and nobody notices until minutes later. We are lucky, as some people lose their loved ones for hours or days. We live with that fear for now. But after the fifth walkout, we decided to set the beep-beep alarm.

It works if Jimmy and I are at home, but it's not a fix when it's just Dad at home. If Dad's hearing aids are not working well, he's on a business call in his office, or blowing leaves on the deck, he doesn't hear the beep-beep alarm. Luckily, on those occasions, the neighbors called him the minute they saw her walking down the street.

"Mr. Myles, she's on the move again," they tell Dad over the phone, and he runs frantically out of the house to find her. He jumps in his van to fetch her as she is far down the street. He pulls alongside and pleads with her to get in. She refuses and keeps walking until she finally gets tired and decides to climb in. Once, she walked into the woods on the street side and just stood there. Dad kept talking to her, and she finally walked to the car.

Jimmy once jumped in the van with Dad when they discovered she had left. They finally found her a quarter mile down our street. When they reached her, Jimmy jumped out and started walking with her.

"Sherry, where are you going?" Jimmy asked her.

"I'm going to the mall!"

"Sherry, it's too far to walk, and it is too hot today to be outside. Let's return to the house, and I will take you to the mall or anywhere you want."

"Okay, but I'm not getting in with him," she said, giving my dad a nasty look.

"I understand."

He walked back to the house with her while my dad drove behind in the van.

"Sit down and let me get you some water. Are you hungry?" Jimmy asked her.

"A little," she replied quietly.

He made turkey sandwiches for both of them and sat with her at the table.

"How's your mom and dad?" she asked him.

"They are fine," he replied.

He didn't try to correct or explain that they were deceased. He just stepped into Mom's reality. And after eating half of her sandwich, she stood up and walked to her room for a nap, forgetting about the mall as quickly as she had forgotten his parents were dead.

When I arrived home, I found Mom and Dad watching the news. They seemed fine. Jimmy was outside smoking a cigar on the back deck and filled me in on the walkout.

"Thank you for being there for her today, and thanks for helping Dad," I said, hugging him.

"I need a long hug today," he said as I tried to pull away. I know dealing with my mother brings up memories of his father, who had Alzheimer's for years.

"Don't you think it's weird my mother has never walked out while I'm here at the house?" I asked him.

I wish I could always be here. Unfortunately, it isn't possible since I'm now working a contract event job. I'm grateful for the work. It gives me a chance to get out of the house and pay some bills—like the credit card for our stuff in storage!

My sisters are afraid Mom will fall into the lake, drown, or disappear into the woods. Shannan begins campaigning to move her into a Memory Care facility every time she walks out of the house.

"I don't think she is ready. Dad isn't ready," I say.

"They will never be ready. We have to do what's best for Mom. Plus, it's a huge strain on Dad, and I'm worried about him!" Shannan says.

The truth is, I'm not ready. How will we put Mom into assisted living? I can't imagine that day. It seems like a nightmare.

We visit local Memory Care units, scratching them off the list one by one. Too expensive and too depressing. We see women and men slumped over in wheelchairs. Please! My mother is not there yet. I hide the Memory Care brochures upstairs on a stool at the foot of my bed, a constant reminder that the end is near. The clock is ticking.

Our housekeeper, Dana, is a fantastic friend to my mom and comes to spend time with her every other week. She takes Mom to lunch and plans activities. She brings crafts, and they sit at the table painting and coloring. Mom adores Dana and is thrilled when she brings her adorable ten-year-old granddaughter, Parker. One day, I found them standing around the kitchen table playing jacks.

"Did you know my mom loved to play jacks?" I ask Dana.

"No, Parker picked them out at the Dollar Tree after lunch today."

I remember sitting on the floor in our kitchen as a kid with Mom teaching us how to flip the jacks in our palms, bounce the ball, and pick up the jacks. She was an expert jacks player while we clumsily tried to play. I remember storming off, frustrated. Incredibly, Mom can still play jacks. I jump in and try to play. We laugh as the ball bounces across the kitchen, and Parker runs to find it.

On one of Dana's visiting days, Dad and I sneak off to meet my sisters at a "Lunch and Learn" at Alzheimer's Services. The staff is lovely, and they inform us of the various resources available, including a Memory Care Day program called Charlie's Place in the building. After lunch, they gave us a tour of the facility, where we saw Alzheimer's patients in various stages, having lunch, crafting, and being entertained by an animated team member.

"This would be great for Mom," Shannan says.

Dad and I agree, but getting her here is our dilemma. They suggest Dad bring her for lunch the following Friday, when they will have a sing-along. Dad drives there, and Mom refuses to get out of the car. He argues with her, but finally, she goes in with him. They see the musician Jack, whom they happen to know. Mom loves the music, sings along, and enjoys lunch. She hugs the sweet team members as they leave.

"We will see you tomorrow," they tell Mom.

"This is so nice," she says.

Dad signs her up for the following Monday.

"Where are we going?" Mom asks when Dad drives her to Charlie's Place.

"Charlie's Place."

"I'm not going there. It's nice, but not for me. I'll let you know when I want to go there."

Discouraged, Dad takes her to lunch instead.

"How did it go?" I asked him that afternoon.

"It didn't," he says, shaking his head and rolling his eyes.

We moved to Plan B—I contacted a senior home care service, and the owner came to the house to meet us. Mom likes him. He has a great personality and claims to have the perfect woman, who will spend four hours with Mom and take her to lunch. Mom seems open to the idea.

Joan, a lovely woman with a big personality, stops by the next day to meet Mom, and they hit it off. They sit and have coffee. Dad hears them chatting and laughing in the living room. We scheduled Joan for four hours the following day. She picks Mom up, and they go to lunch, then return to the house to watch TV. She plans to come back next week, but after she leaves, Mom tells Dad she doesn't need a babysitter. We canceled the next visit with the service. We are back to square one.

We are hitting the wall. We are beat. I try to work out of the house several times weekly, but it's too distracting.

It's Monday, a typical "red beans and rice" dinner night in Louisiana. I fix Mom's tuna salad for lunch, and she sits eating at the counter, watching me chop onions, celery, garlic, green onions, and bell peppers for the beans. I sauté the diced ham and smoked sausage and add the red beans, which had soaked overnight. I throw everything in a big pot with store-bought chicken stock and lots of Creole seasoning, salt, and pepper. Soon, the house smells delicious. I prepare a big green salad. Mom takes a nap while I watch my beans simmer all afternoon and work on my laptop at the kitchen table.

At 5:30, we have an early-bird dinner, and all is well. The red beans and rice are delicious. Dad, Jimmy, and I inhale them, and Mom barely picks at hers. We serve her dinner now on a small plate. She can't handle big plates. It's too confusing and causes her extreme anxiety.

At the end of dinner, I bring Mom her pills in a small bowl.

"What's this for?" she asks.

"It's your medicine, Sherry," Dad blurts out.

"Here, Mom, let me help you," I say, trying to hand her one pill at a time while holding a glass of water. She turns her face away.

"Not this again. You take them," Mom exclaims, pouting.

"Sherry, take the pills!" Dad demands.

It escalates, and before you know it, she is screaming, Dad is screaming, and I'm shaking—all over a bunch of damn pills. My "drama-queen, frick it, I'm done" trigger explodes.

"I have to get out of here. I can't deal with this tonight," I tell Jimmy, grabbing my purse off the counter and storming out the door. He grabs his keys from the counter and follows me.

"Let's go see a movie. I need a distraction," I say, crying as I pull out my phone and look at the film schedule.

We are halfway to the movie theater and my cell phone rings. It's Dad.

"Well, she did it this time! You need to come back now!" he yells.

"What's happening, Dad?" I panic, and my heart feels like it's going to jump out of my chest.

"She walked out of the house, telling me she was going to tell the neighbors that I'm abusing her and have them call the police."

"We're turning around now. Where are you?"

"I'm down the street. I followed her, she went to a stranger's front door and knocked on their door."

"Oh, my God! What house? Jimmy, hurry!" I scream.

"A house way down the street. The people who live there opened the door and let her in. I'm standing here on the street outside their yard. I guess the police will arrive at any moment to arrest me. What a mess! This is awful," Dad says.

"Dad, that's ridiculous! Knock on their door. We are on our way back."

Mom ran away and went into a stranger's house. I texted my sisters.

OMG! Rob and I are on our way! Shannan texts back.

"A man is coming out of the house and walking toward me. Let me go talk to him," Dad says and hangs up.

Ten minutes later, we drove down the street and see Mom and Dad walking to our driveway. Dad is following her. She walks up the driveway to the back door and goes inside. I jump out of the car and run in after her.

"Mom, are you Okay?"

"Yes, I'm fine. I went to visit my friends," she says, walking to the living room. She sits calmly at the end of the old green sofa and starts watching *The Voice.* I follow her.

"Well, that's nice. Can I get you a glass of water?" I ask.

"Sure."

I head back to the kitchen to get a glass of water and see Dad and Jimmy outside, talking on the driveway as Shannan and Rob drive up. Shannan jumps out of her car and rushes into the house. I hand her the glass of water.

"Bring this to Mom in the living room while I talk to Dad."

She grabs the glass, rolls her eyes, and shakes her head at me.

"Hi, Mom. Rob and I came to visit," she says as I walk out the back door.

Rob is now standing with the guys, shaking his head as Dad tells him the story. I join them and interrupt.

"Are you okay, Dad? Did the police come?" I blurt out, cutting him off.

"No. She didn't ask them to call the police. She just knocked on their door. She was out of breath and asked if she could have a glass of water. She sat down in a chair and told them, 'He is following me.'"

They looked out the window and saw me standing on the street. The homeowner, Larry, came to speak with me. I told him she has Alzheimer's, and he said they figured it out—his mother-in-law had Alzheimer's, and they are familiar with this behavior.

His wife came out the front door with Mom, and Mom started walking home. She wouldn't look at me, so I just followed her home."

"This is crazy, Dad! I'm so sorry we left you," I said.

"I need a drink!" Dad exclaims.

"Of course you do! I'll get it," Rob says.

We file into the house, and Rob goes to the refrigerator, pulling out Dad's big bottle of Chardonnay from the door. He opens it. I pull out wineglasses for them.

"Shannan, do you want a glass of wine?" I call out from the kitchen.

"Sure!" she yells from the living room.

"I think I would rather have a whiskey," Dad tells Rob.

"Now you're talking!" Rob pulls a bottle from Dad's bar.

Soon they both have whiskey on the rocks and go to the living room. Jimmy just shakes his head at me and starts cleaning the kitchen.

"How are you doing, Sherry?" Rob asks as he leans down to kiss Mom on the cheek.

"I'm fine. I'm glad y'all came to visit," Mom says, smiling at Rob.

"Yes, this is a surprise!" Dad says and swigs his whiskey.

"Are y'all hungry? Want some red beans?" I ask them.

"No, we just finished eating. Thanks," Shannan replies and continues to tell Mom about the kids. Rob and Dad chat as if it's just another friendly family visit. I can't sit still. I head to the kitchen to help Jimmy clean in silence. I want to scream, This isn't happening, right? But it is happening and just getting worse by the day.

I walk out with Shannan and Rob as they leave.

"Thank you for coming to help!" I say, hugging her.

"It's time, Peg. It's only going to get worse," she tells me.

"I know," and we both shake our heads with tears in our eyes.

I watch them drive away, then I turn to walk back into the house, but change my mind. I quickly turned around and headed down the path to the lake.

I sit on a bench. The sun is going down, and it is a magnificent evening. The stillness of the lake and the colors of the sky reflecting on the water are a picture of serenity— the complete opposite of what I feel in my heart, mind, body, and soul. I'm all alone here. Alone in my grief, my confusion, and my anger.

"Why, God, why?" I cry out loud, and then I sob. I cry until there are no more tears. It's now twilight, and the moon is over the lake.

I receive no reply from God tonight, so I turn and walk away.

Mom's Red Beans and Rice

Ingredients:

1 pound pack of dried red kidney beans
One ham bone or ham hock (optional)
1-2 cups of chopped ham (best if from a leftover baked ham, but can use diced packaged ham, not sliced)
One pound of smoked sausage, cut into one-inch pieces.
3 Tbsp. butter
2 medium onions, chopped
1 bell pepper, chopped
3 stalks of celery, chopped
2 garlic pods, chopped
½ bunch of green onions chopped fine
½ cup of chopped parsley
2 Bay leaves
4 cups of water
4 cups of chicken broth
Salt, Pepper, and Cajun seasoning

Instructions:

Rinse beans and soak in water overnight.
Drain beans and place them with ham in a large pot with water/chicken broth to cover.
If you have a ham bone, put the whole bone in the pot.
Bring beans to boil.
In a separate pan, brown sausage on medium-high heat, then drain on a plate covered with a paper towel.
Drain excess fat from the bottom of the pan and add butter and vegetables. Sauté until soft.
Add Bay leaves to the beans, along with the vegetables and sausage.
Bring to a rolling boil for 30 minutes, stirring every few minutes.

219

Reduce the heat to a simmer for one to two hours, or until the beans are tender. Add additional water or chicken broth as needed.

Stir frequently to prevent the beans from sticking to the bottom of the pan.

When the beans are tender, use a large spoon to smash some of them to the side of the pot to make the beans creamy

Taste and add salt, pepper, and Cajun seasoning to taste.

Yield:

8 servings

Serve red beans over white rice with green salad or coleslaw, hot French bread, and hot sauce on the side.

CHAPTER TWELVE
BROKEN ORNAMENTS &
BROKEN HEARTS

"Alexa, play Christmas music," I say, and Barbra Streisand's "O Holy Night" begins.

"This makes me cry," Mom says.

"Me too, Mom. We need something more upbeat today."

"Alexa, play '50s Christmas music," I add, and "Jingle Bell Rock" kicks in—a better choice.

This holiday season will probably be Mom's last Christmas at home, and I'm not feeling the spirit. I'm putting on my best "let's have fun decorating for Christmas" face, determined to make the day festive.

This morning, Dad and Jimmy brought the decorations down from the attic. The living room is filled with plastic crates, big boxes, and sections of the fake tree. The fresh trees of my childhood were replaced long ago by this pre-lit one—except only half the lights are working, so Jimmy ran out for more white lights while Dad began assembling.

Growing up, we had colored twinkle lights that "danced" to the holiday music. Jimmy's New York family used white lights. That led to an argument during our first year of marriage in New Orleans.

"I want colored twinkle lights," I said as we picked out our first tree at the Christmas tree lot.

"That's tacky and childish. White lights are classier," Jimmy declared.

He won the light battle. I told my friend Jackie about our light disagreement.

"I always have colored twinkle lights! Those New Yorkers just don't get it," she laughed—and gifted us a box of colored lights at a pre-Christmas dinner. Jimmy shook his head while we were cackling. I went home and wrapped the colored lights around our Ficus plant—a twinkling compromise.

Soon it's just Mom and me in the living room. Dad retreats to his upstairs office; Jimmy disappears to smoke a cigar. They both believe decorating is for the ladies. It's strange how much has changed. During our first year back in Louisiana, Mom directed me on where every ornament should go. Last year, she lasted ten minutes and didn't care where I hung them. Now she just sits and watches. Her ornaments, still in their original boxes, are beautiful. After thirty minutes, she walks out without a word and goes to her room. I wish I'd asked my sisters to help, but they're busy decorating their own trees.

Despite the twinkling branches and bright colors, the sadness of this Christmas fills the room. I thought this would help. It doesn't. The joy of Christmas doesn't live here anymore.

"Alexa, play Barbra Streisand Christmas," I say, and "Silent Night" comes on. I hang ornaments alone with tears streaming, aching for Christmases past.

***

"Daddy, take a picture of just me!" I announce, posing with one hand on my hip and the other touching my homemade stocking—my name glittering in red.

"I hate this granny cap. It's dumb. Why do we have to wear these? I hate taking pictures!" Shannan complains.

"Where did Erin go?" Mom asks, irritated, as she heads down the hall to find her jumping on the bed or tumbling down the hallway.

"Oh no, Kelly, now is not the time to eat candy canes! It's all over your nightgown and in your hair," Mom scolds, snapping the peppermint stick away and wiping her down.

We're in the formal living room, gathered around a cardboard fireplace with a spinning light behind a cutout log to mimic a roaring fire. All four little Sweeney sisters wear flannel granny nightgowns with matching caps in red and green. We're obsessed with the new "fireplace." Our decor grew every year, and the faux hearth was a welcome addition to our Wilton Drive house, which had no real fireplace. Our stockings were hung by the chimney with care, and we believed Santa would come down through the chimney. We'd lie on the floor and peer up the chute. We believed in the magic of Christmas!

Mom staged us while Dad snapped the pictures— maybe our first official photo-card shoot. We've all shared it on Facebook in recent years. It looks adorable—no hint of the inevitable family drama. But there was always drama with four Southern daughters and their mother. Mom would be totally outdone, stressed, and fussing at poor Dad and at us.

"This is like pulling teeth! No one is listening to me!" she'd exclaim. No one was having fun during the shoot. Somehow, we always managed to capture one perfect picture to mail to relatives, friends, and Dad's business associates, along with his annual letter.

The photo backdrops changed over the years—lined on the stairs from oldest to youngest; in front of the flocked tree; in front of the new house; with our pet pony, Ginger, in the backyard; roasting marshmallows by the fire pit; and once on Thanksgiving vacation in the Smokies. As we grew older, Mom and Dad joined the frame. A family friend—or our grandmother—took the pictures. Once, we even hired a photographer who posed us on the trunk of a big oak tree; that one was enlarged, framed, and hung in their bedroom. I was a college freshman, laughing now at my Dorothy Hamill haircut, jean skirt, and sweater vest—my preppy sorority look.

One year, Mom made a giant green-foil cutout Christmas tree to hang on the wall, filled with our past photo cards—oldest at the top. I wonder what happened to that treasure.

We each had a personal ornament box, our names scrawled in red. The first Sunday of December, we'd go to Heroman's holiday open house—the official kick-off. We wore our church outfits to Mass and raced to the noon opening. The store was packed. We'd snake through aisles, eyes wide, choosing one new ornament for our boxes.

"Do you like this one, Mama?" we'd ask—needing her approval. Of course, she checked the price.

She'd nod or suggest another while we nibbled free star butter cookies dusted with red and green sprinkles and sipped hot chocolate.

My ornament box traveled with me to Houston, New York, New Orleans, and Los Angeles. It lives now in storage with the rest of our stuff. For years, we spent the holidays with my family in Louisiana or Jimmy's in New York, so we often skipped trees in tiny apartments. Later, when we didn't always fly "home," I needed our own tree. I'd open my childhood box first—those scrappy, beloved ornaments— before the prettier adult collection. The old ones weren't sophisticated, but they were mine. I hung them in the back by the wall. I knew they were there. That was enough.

Our Christmas Eve parties growing up were epic—an open house from 7:00–10:00 p.m. The house overflowed with neighbors, friends, and relatives, laughter spilling from the kitchen into the living room. The tradition began when I was in grade school. We would all be dressed in our velvet dresses, white tights, and patent leather shoes, posing for a quick picture before piling into the station wagon for the packed 4:30 p.m. Mass at St. Thomas Moore. The scent of incense clung to us as we flew out of the church and rushed home to get ready for the party!

Mom's food stretched across the dining table and buffet: hot Crabmeat Mornay dip, meatballs, ham, roast beef, spinach dip, cheese and fruit boards, and more. The kitchen table was set with dessert—cookies, pies, cakes. Guests brought dishes; there was food for an army. Dad turned the laundry room into a bar by laying plywood over the washer and dryer and draping a white cloth—whiskey, scotch, rum, vodka, ice chests of beer, wine, and sodas on the floor. Our neighbor Angelle played piano while we caroled.

Mom—perfect Southern hostess—handed out song sheets and sang at the piano, positively glowing. She loved to sing and always said that in her next life she wanted to come back as Barbra Streisand.

As we got married and had babies, the guest list shifted to family plus a few close friends. The centerpiece became our homemade nativity play directed by Mom and starring the grandchildren. The girls rotated as Mary, the boys as Joseph. The first year, five-year-old Caroline was Mary, and three-year-old Myles—named for Dad—was Joseph. Caroline tucked a baby doll under Mom's blue robe and, at "and the baby Jesus was born," pulled him out and cradled him. We cheered. She beamed.

The following year, we had a real baby for Jesus, and from then on, the newest baby got the role. Kelly could hardly wait to have children so that hers could be Jesus, Mary, and Joseph. Friends' children were angels with fake candles. It was quite a production.

Mom relished being director, producer, set designer, and stage manager. The grandkids came the week before to rehearse and build cardboard sets. On Christmas Eve, she spread costumes across her king-size bed. I was assistant director—dressing kids and lining them up in the living room. One year, I sang "Hard Candy Christmas" with them, and the guys teased that I was stealing the show.

The nativity ended with "Silent Night," then they made a quick costume change into elf outfits. A grandson playing Santa burst in with "Ho, ho, ho!" dragging a sack while the others rang gold handbells and sang "Jingle Bells." Santa handed out gifts: all the women got candles or ornaments labeled "Lady," and the "Man" gift was always socks. Running joke. Jimmy or a brother-in-law would deadpan, "I wonder what this is," as they unwrapped socks.

Soon, the kids changed into pajamas, leaving costumes in a heap. They couldn't wait to get home before the real Santa arrived. Jimmy and Dad cleaned the kitchen while I helped Mom pack costumes. When the house finally quieted, the four of us sat in the living room, watching the lights dance and listening to music. That was the sweet spot. Mom would talk about how precious her grandchildren were and how much fun she'd had. I forgot the stress and just soaked her in.

Slowly, before any diagnosis, her anxiety grew. She began snapping at us—insisting we weren't helping, even as we ran ourselves ragged. Even her famous macaroni and cheese became too much. We pared the spread down, starting with cheese and crackers, followed by dinner. Dad picked up Honey Baked ham and turkey; my sisters brought sides; the grandkids made cookies. After one last drama-filled Christmas Eve, we called it quits.

"Mom can't handle hosting anymore. We need to rethink Christmas Eve," Shannan said—the voice of reason.

"I'll book a big table at a restaurant after Mass," she decided.

Mom pushed back, but Shannan persuaded her. Dad agreed wholeheartedly. And just like that, a lifetime of Christmas Eves moved into the memory files.

"We won't be able to come to Baton Rouge this year," I told them. "Christmas is midweek, and Jimmy can't get off work."

Deep down, I was relieved to miss the "first restaurant Christmas Eve." It felt wrong—cold—not a "Sweeney Christmas Eve." I pictured Mom and Dad returning to a quiet house, just the two of them.

While my sisters set the new plan, Jimmy and I planned our own Christmas in Los Angeles. We'd always wanted to attend Christmas Eve Mass at the chapel at Serra Retreat Center in Malibu—perched on a high cliff over the Pacific. Traffic would be a pain from the Valley, but we were determined.

We discovered Serra after reading a *Los Angeles Magazine* piece about Frank Sinatra after his death. It described the beautiful grounds of Serra and how he loved to walk there. The first time we drove up the winding road, it took our breath away. We brought visiting friends and family there over the years—including both sets of parents, one Thanksgiving. There's a photo of the six of us, smiling with Malibu beneath us.

While my family went to Mass and then to Ruffino's in Baton Rouge, Jimmy and I arrived at Serra with time to stroll the grounds. We stood at the cliff's edge as the sun sank—orange, deep blue, purple, pink—the colors of my magical childhood tree.

"Spectacular, spectacular," Jimmy said.

"Beyond spectacular," I agreed, moving closer in the cold. Arms wrapped tight, we watched the sky burn out. We didn't know it would be our last time at Serra—or our last L.A. Christmas—but in that moment, we were simply grateful.

"Merry Christmas, Jimmy Dean," I murmured.

"Merry Christmas, Peggy Bug," he said, and we kissed before heading to the chapel.

Mass was lovely. The friends-and-family crowd included Malibu neighbors: Martin Sheen and Dick Van

Dyke, both doing readings. Afterward, Father Warren invited everyone for hot apple cider and cookies. I grew up on *Mary Poppins* and *Chitty Chitty Bang Bang*, so meeting Dick Van Dyke over a tray of cookies felt like a dream—he was as gracious as you'd imagine.

By the time we got back to the Valley, it was after 9:00 p.m. and everything was closed, so we heated a can of Progresso chicken noodle soup. We laughed at our "holiday meal," turned on the tree lights, and put on Christmas music. We ate soup from coffee mugs, opened our gifts, and then, to the Rat Pack singing "White Christmas," Jimmy pulled me up and we danced in the living room.

Back in Louisiana, the reports were good. The restaurant dinner was a hit. They even rented a shuttle to drive around to look at the lights afterward, and Mom loved it. When we moved back the next year, we rolled with the new plan.

Which brings me to now: alone, finishing the tree for what will probably be Mom's last Christmas at home. I stack the empty ornament boxes and slide them aside.

Mom and Dad no longer buy presents for everyone, and I haven't had time to shop. The space beneath the tree is bare except for a manger sitting on the red tree skirt Mom sewed years ago. Once upon a time, you could barely find a specific gift under the mountain of beautifully wrapped gifts. Now we draw names. Everything is pared down.

On December 23, I venture out to pick up a few simple gifts, wrap them, and set them under the tree. Better than nothing.

That night, we went with my sister Erin's family to a huge Christian church—rock band, pro-quality choir, giant screens, breathtaking visuals. They pass out candles at the door. Near the end, the lights drop and the ushers light the end of each row. Flame by flame, the room glows. I snap a photo of Mom with her candle, her face lit like a lantern—radiant, singing "O Come, All Ye Faithful." My heart nearly bursts.

We take a family photo by the giant outdoor tree and head home: one service down, one to go. Our two-day holiday has now become three.

On Christmas Eve, Mom lets me select her clothes and help her shower. I do her hair and makeup. She looks festive in black velvet pants and a sparkly red twinset with pearls sewn into the collar.

"Where are we going?" she asks.

"Mass with the girls, then out to dinner."

We meet Kelly, Shannan, and their families at their Catholic church, then have a lingering dinner at French Market Bistro. We feast on platters of charbroiled oysters topped with crabmeat, butter, garlic, and Parmesan; steaming bowls of crab-and-brie bisque; salads; and hot French bread. Prime rib and trout almondine for entrées. Decadent white-chocolate bread pudding for dessert. A Christmas Eve to remember!

We no longer dream about Honey Baked Ham and mac and cheese. No all-day prep, no epic cleanup—and no drama. We laugh, enjoy each other, and savor the Creole food. It's easy and festive. The girls order a mimosa for Mom. She drinks half, and the fizz makes her giddy. She's happy. Everyone glows.

As hard as it was to release our old traditions, I relish our new "keep it simple" Christmas Eve. There's still plenty that glitters.

On Christmas morning, my parents, Jimmy, and I open presents. I cook eggs, bacon, fresh fruit, and hot cinnamon rolls. Mom and I watch *White Christmas* and stand to dance to "Sisters." Then it's off to the family afternoon gumbo-and-gifts tradition—blue jeans, holiday sweaters, and, of course, my red cowboy boots.

We swapped presents and appetizers, then dove into Scott's chicken-and-sausage gumbo with Nanny's potato salad, Shannan's special green sensation salad, hot, crusty French bread, and platters of the grandkids' cookies and fudge.

Mom soaks up attention, especially from her grandchildren. Does anyone else think this could be our last Christmas with her?

I look around and feel the blessing. We're twenty-one now. Everyone is laughing, talking over each other, and snapping photos.

"Think we should take the tree down?" Dad asks a few days later.

"Not yet, Dad. Mom loves the tree. Let's leave it a few more days," I say—knowing that once it's gone, Christmas with my mother is over.

New Year's passes. It's January 2nd, and it's finally time. Mom watches as I begin taking ornaments down. She stands to "help," but it's all backward. I place ornaments in their boxes; she takes them out and puts them back on the tree—or piles them on the coffee table—Alzheimer's insanity. My nerves are frayed.

"Mom, what are you doing?"

"I'm putting the ornaments away."

"No, Mom, I'm putting them away. You're taking them out of the boxes."

"Stop yelling at me!"

"I'm not yelling," I say—and then drop one of her favorites.

"Look what you did! You need to be more careful," she scolds.

Right then, another beloved ornament slips from a branch and shatters.

"You never cared about my things," she yells.

I lost it and stormed upstairs. Jimmy meets me at the landing.

"What's going on down there?"

"I can't deal with it. I'm done," I sob, and slam our door.

Jimmy goes downstairs and quietly starts packing the tree. Every time he turns around, she pulls ornaments back out of their boxes.

"Sherry, I've got this," he says gently. "Why don't you take a nap, and I'll come get you in a little while?"

She wanders off. Later, Jimmy admits he didn't bother matching each ornament to its "right" box. He was done—with all of it, including me.

By the time I come out, Dad and Jimmy are loading boxes into the attic. I carry a few up to the door. Soon, it's all packed away. Dad closes the attic door. Christmas is over.

A week later, I noticed the little pillows spelling N O E L still on the dormer window, and a plaid bow Mom tied to the lamp beside her spot on the sofa. I left them. They may be the last remnants of Christmas with my mother.

Christmas was always her favorite. She gave birth to it in our home and in our hearts. But our producer, director, set designer, and stage manager left us years ago. This year, she was just a visitor, going along with our program. And although we found lovely moments, it wasn't what it used to be. It will never be what it used to be.

I can't imagine Christmas without my mother. The magic has gone—faded like old photo Christmas cards and shattered into little pieces, just like her broken ornaments and our broken hearts.

Mom's Mac-N-Cheese

Ingredients:

16-ounce package of elbow macaroni
2 eggs
½ Tbsp. sugar
salt and pepper to taste
1 12-ounce can of evaporated milk
1 cup of whole milk
2 16-ounce bags of mild or sharp grated cheese
1 stick of salted butter, melted

Instructions:

Preheat oven to 350°F
Cook macaroni in salted boiling water until tender, then drain well in a colander.
Beat eggs and sugar together in a small bowl.
Add evaporated and whole milk to eggs.
Mix macaroni, butter, and one package of cheese.
Add the egg/milk mixture and place it in a buttered baking dish.
Cover with more cheese and bake at 350°F degrees for 45 minutes with a tented aluminum foil cover. Remove the foil from the dish for the last 5 minutes to let the top cheese become toasty.
Double the recipe if needed.

Yield:

Serves 8-12 on a buffet

Family Notes:

Growing up, my baby sister Kelly lived on Kraft macaroni and cheese from the box. It was all she ate besides milk and candy. (And she became the doctor in our family!) When the grandkids were young, my mother began making homemade mac and cheese for her precious grandkids. However, it was a massive hit with the brothers-in-law. She would make a double batch, and they would scoop up leftovers to take home. We always said, "Mom is making the mac and cheese for the grandkids," but we knew we were all going to indulge in the cheesy yumminess. Now we divide up the family favorites, and everyone has had a chance to make Mom's mac and cheese. It is always a big hit!

CHAPTER THIRTEEN
LEAVING THE NEST

"Peggy, come see," Mom yelled up the stairs. "We have a bird's nest!"

"Amazing!" I exclaimed as we stood together, peering through the window at the bird's nest built by a cute little yellow bird.

"I love it. What a wonderful gift!" Mom told Erin when she opened her Mother's Day present last May. She pulled out a wooden rustic birdhouse with a clear plastic back.

"It attaches to the window with the suction cups. You can watch the birds make their nest, see them lay eggs, hatch the eggs, and then fly away," Erin explained.

"How cool," I said as Dad took the birdhouse outside and set it on our window in the hallway between the kitchen and the living room. It was perfect!

We peeked several times a day through the peek-a-boo window of our birdhouse and saw the mama bird sitting on her nest. Sometimes it sensed us and flew away.

"Aww, I think we scared her," Mom said as our little bird flew away.

"She will be back soon, Mom," I assured her.

"I think it's a Goldfinch," Dad said to us.

I looked up the spiritual meaning of Goldfinch on the internet and found that it represents positivity, optimism, and the value of happiness, joy, and simplicity in life. How timely! It was a guidepost I needed for my life: Find joy and happiness each day. Keep it simple. Celebrate life. Our little yellow bird shared life lessons with us, and we were blessed.

A few weeks later, we spotted the newly laid eggs, which were pure magic. They were small, pretty, and looked like miniature marbleized Easter eggs. We were fascinated that some eggs were different colors. Our cute mama bird sat patiently, warming her eggs, ready to hatch.

"Peggy, they are here!" Mom happily shrieked one morning. I ran down the stairs and met her at the peek-a-boo window.

"Look how adorable they are," I said as we stood mesmerized, watching the five baby birds open and close their mouths, waiting for their mama to feed them and bring them nourishment. She soon appeared with worms to feed her babies. It was a first-hand look at life inside a birdhouse, and the joy it brought to my mother was priceless. She watched life happen as hers slipped away.

Come see our baby birds. I texted my sisters and sent them pictures.

Erin came over with my niece, Peyton. They were as excited as we were.

"They are precious," Erin exclaimed.

"So precious!" Mom said with a huge smile on her face.

"Simply precious," I chimed in.

Jimmy laughed, watching us.

"There it is again, the P-word. Your Mama and your sisters always say, 'They are so precious.' The difference between y'all and my New York sisters is they would say they are just too frickin cute!" he told us.

"Jimmy!" Mom scolded him, laughing.

A week later, I was sitting with Mom eating breakfast, and I glimpsed our mama bird flying around the birdhouse. I turned to see one of the baby birds fly out and drop to the ground briefly before taking off, flapping its wings and going airborne within seconds.

"Look, Mom, they're flying!"

We watched in awe until all the baby birds had flown away. The mama bird flew away after the last one. It was a magical moment of nature, and we could have missed it in seconds.

"We saw the baby birds fly away," Mom announced over and over again that day. Her eyes are animated and filled with joy. The little yellow bird brought us much-needed optimism for a few weeks.

The birdhouse, now void of life, was emptied in the backyard by Dad and placed back on the window. A few months later, the process began again, but one of the baby birds died. We watch his lifeless body in the nest with the other birds. The mama bird must have removed it because the dead bird disappeared one morning. Days later, they were all gone. Did they all die, or did the others fly away? We will never know.

"It's so sad," Mom said with tears.

"I know, Mom," I said, hugging her.

"Jimmy, can you take the birdhouse down and clean it with soap? If there is some type of disease lingering in it, I don't want another bird to nest there," I told him.

He took it down, cleaned it, and set it on the side of the carport to dry. We forgot to place it back on the window. The birdhouse, which brought us simple joy, never went up again.

I think about our sweet birdhouse as the days get harder. We forgot the small stuff that brought Mom so much joy and pleasure—the Scrabble games, the adult coloring books, and the puzzles we made, the walks to the lake to watch the ducks, and our much-loved birdhouse. Our life at home in Louisiana gets smaller and smaller, drearier and drearier, sadder and sadder. Our grief permeates the house like a fog, making it hard to breathe. The hope of life emptied just like the mama bird cleared out her nest—a metaphor for what's to come.

"Dad and I met with the Memory Care director today. They have a one-bedroom available with a private bathroom. The move-in date will be the last Sunday in January," Shannan tells me over the phone in mid-January.

"OK," I say, barely breathing. It's only two weeks away.

"Can you be in charge of packing her clothes?" she asked me.

"Sure, I say," choking back tears.

"Rob and I are going to look at the furniture we have in storage. She will need a double bed, dresser, nightstand, and chairs. Kelly is going to order new bedding and towels. Erin will check what she has. We all need to gather framed pictures, photo albums, and artwork. We need to make it homey and pretty.

It seems so final, and despite knowing we are doing the right thing, it still feels wrong.

The week before, I came home to find Dad sitting in his chair and Mom locked away in her bedroom.

"How was your day?" I asked Dad.

"The worst day ever," he said sadly.

"What happened, Dad?"

"She wanted to leave. She told me this isn't our house and said I'm lying to her. The more I told her this was our house and that we lived here, the more upset she became. She picked up the fireplace shovel and threatened to hit me over the head with it if I didn't stop lying to her."

"Dad, she could kill you with the shovel! What if you had been napping? You wouldn't be able to defend yourself!"

"I know. She held onto it all day—walking in and out of the living room. I didn't know what to do. I just don't know what to do anymore," he tells me with a desperation I have never seen before.

Recently, Mom started believing this wasn't her home. Dad would pull into the driveway after taking her to lunch or for a ride, and she would refuse to get out of the car.

"This isn't my house!" she would say defiantly.

Dad would sit in the van trying to convince her. Finally, frustrated, he would go into the house, waiting and watching her from the kitchen. Eventually, she would come shuffling in, calling him names and telling him she hated him before going to their bedroom and locking the door.

She pulled me aside one evening and said, "Peggy, I'm worried. The people who live here will be upset that we are living here in their house."

I tried to explain to her that we lived here, pointing out her clothing, pictures, jewelry, and rosary beads, but she just didn't get it. It is now a strange house to her—her dream house, the house she loved from the minute she set foot in it, the house she had spent so much time decorating over the years. It is as unfamiliar as the room she will be moving into at the Memory Care unit.

I can't begin to imagine what it is like for her to be living in a strange house. If I woke up one day in a strange house, I would be filled with anxiety, anger, and sadness. It would be a nightmare that never ends.

"Where'd my mother go? She was just here!" she said to me one night while we sat on the old green couch watching television.

"Where did my brother go? He was here a minute ago," she told me another night.

"Where are the little girls? They were just here playing with me," she said to Dad one night.

I wonder if Alzheimer's is making her delusional, or maybe they are here in spirit. I like to believe that Nanny, Poppy, and Uncle Bubby are here with her. Their ghosts ease her pain and confusion, paving the way for her to cross to the other side. I imagine them holding her hand, sitting with her in the living room, lying on the bed while she naps, whispering to her, "You are going to be alright. We can do this together."

I imagine the "little children" as angels paving her way, or maybe she sees us, her precious daughters, as children. Are we playing with our dolls? Are we baking in our Easy Bake Oven, bringing her our little cakes and pies? Am I dressing up in my dance review costumes and putting on a show for her?

Her mother died twenty years ago, but her brother died just last year. Mom had already been diagnosed with Alzheimer's when my dad received the call. Hammet Murphy, or Uncle Bubby, as we called him, lived in Sweden and had a massive stroke. When his wife arrived home from work, she found him unconscious on the bedroom floor. The diagnosis was not good.

Mom told Dad she wanted to see her brother before he died. Dad scrambled to find airline tickets, and off they went to Sweden. We didn't think it was a good idea for an Alzheimer's patient to travel internationally, but looking back, I'm grateful she could be by her brother's side.

Uncle Bubby never regained consciousness, but Mom spoke to him, hugged and kissed him, held his hand, and loved him. His daughter, Leyla, played YouTube videos of New Orleans rainfall because he loved the rainstorms in his hometown. On that Friday, they pulled the plug, and my Uncle Bubby slipped away. I know my grandmother was there to bring him home to heaven.

My nephew Myles flew in from Prague to be with my parents in Stockholm that weekend, and Bubby's other daughter, Siobhan, flew in from Boston. They celebrated his life with a lovely dinner the night before they left, and my dad told each of them that Mom had Alzheimer's.

When they arrived back in Louisiana, she seemed quiet and sad for a few days, but I think she had forgotten he had died by the following week. I wonder if losing her only sibling accelerated her Alzheimer's.

Can emotional pain drain your brain? I feel like my brain is being hammered from watching my mother slip away. I can't imagine losing a sibling with or without Alzheimer's. My respect for my dad for bringing Mom across the world to sit by her brother's side as he slipped away is tremendous. My father would do anything for his family. I know this to be true at the deepest level. The thought of Dad being hurt by Mom with the fireplace shovel is more than I can bear. Losing her to the Alzheimer's battle is unbearable. But if I lost my father because of her Alzheimer's, from stress, or being hit by the shovel, it would shake me to my core. I could never come back from losing him and her to Alzheimer's at the same time.

I needed to tell my sisters about the shovel incident. Part of me wanted to keep it a secret because I knew this would be the last straw.

I went to check on Mom first and found her bedroom door locked. This time, I didn't have the energy to plead with her to open it or to reach for the key on top of the door jam. Instead, I walked upstairs to our room. I sat on the bed and texted my sisters about the shovel incident, hesitating to hit SEND as I knew I would pull the trigger on Memory Care.

It's time, Peggy, I heard in my head. I pushed SEND, then lay down on the bed and sobbed. I hate this fricken disease. Screw you, Alzheimer's. You have sucked the soul out of us!

I pulled the trigger on Mom's Memory Care sentence, and within twenty-four hours, she was registered, a deposit paid, and she is stamped with an invisible due date. My beautiful and loving mother is signed, sealed, and ready to be delivered to a locked-down Memory Care unit at a local assisted living facility.

I look at the calendar on my iPhone and count the days before moving her into Memory Care. There are thirteen days, including two weekends. The countdown has begun. I try to stay in the moment, concentrate on my task, and pack her things.

I look in Mom's closet on Saturday morning after Kelly picks her up to take her to lunch. For the last year, her closet has become my focus whenever she is out of the house. I storm through her closet and bathroom cabinets, looking under the bed and the furniture for soiled clothes. She is having accidents and hiding her clothes. I follow my nose. I wash clothes and towels, clean bathrooms, and wipe down closets. She no longer places the hangers on the closet rod. She hangs them on other clothing hangers facing outwards. They get heavy and fall in heaps to the ground.

"Can you please organize her side of the closet? It's a real mess," Dad has said to me more than once.

"I did, Dad, but she messed it up a few days later. Mom has to look at her clothes this way. I think it's easier for her brain," I explained.

"You're right," he replies.

For the past year, I have rotated her clothes to the front of the closet, so she doesn't wear the same thing over and over, pulling out matching tops with pants and placing them together. Sometimes it works, but I usually find them thrown at the back of the closet. She wears the same outfit repeatedly. It makes no sense to me, but it makes perfect sense in her world—the easier, softer way for her depleted, shriveled brain.

Life doesn't make any sense these days. I feel like I live in a carnival fun house.

I fight with her twice a week to take a shower. She claims to have taken a shower, but there are no washcloths or towels to prove it. Additionally, she is still wearing the same clothes from the last two days and has a noticeable smell. Shower time is a nightmare. She fights me every minute. I'm practically standing in the shower stall with her and getting soaked.

"Do you get your kicks out of this?" she says bitterly as I get her to turn around and wash her backside. I know my mom changed my diaper, but this is the hardest thing I've ever done. I hand her a clean, soaped-up washcloth to wash because I can't make myself violate her privacy face-to-face. She is furious with the process and continues to tell me so. I know she feels better once she has showered, and she definitely smells better.

"Don't you feel great, Mom? A nice hot shower always makes me feel better."

"Humph," is all she says. I'm the bad guy here. She hates me. I'm trying to help her, and it only makes her angry.

Most of the time, I walk out of the bathroom exhausted and angry. I walk up the stairs, and Jimmy usually meets me with a big hug.

"That sounded rough," he says, holding me tight while he lets me cry.

Shannan calls with my move-out instructions.

"Go to the mall, Peg, and buy her some pants and simple tops. She also needs nightgowns or pajamas, as they have to change out of their clothes every night."

Good luck with that, I think, as she hasn't worn nightgowns in years. I gave up the pajama fight a long time ago.

Since spending money on new clothes doesn't make sense, I head to our favorite Goodwill. Memory Care recommends pull-up pants and shirts that can be easily washed and folded. I filled a shopping cart with elastic-waist pants in black, navy, khaki, and pink. I peruse the "Women's Shirts" racks and find colorful tops from her favorite designers. I throw in nightgowns and pajamas. Everything is $3.99. I walk out with two huge plastic bags, then drive to Walmart to buy large packs of underwear, bras, and toiletries.

Will she realize these aren't her clothes? Will she like them? I think she may like some of them, but it brings me little comfort. I feel like an imposter setting in motion the grand plan.

I wash, fold, and pack everything in secret suitcases hidden upstairs in the guest bedroom late at night after she has gone to bed. Out of sight, out of mind. Not! The move-out suitcases are out of her sight, but not out of my mind, and are a constant reminder of my limited time living with my mother.

It feels like the biggest betrayal, and I know she will never forgive me. I feel guilty and ashamed for doing this behind her back. It has to be the lowest of lows. I tell myself repeatedly that it is for the best. She will live in a safe place with a staff trained to take care of her, but it doesn't bring me comfort.

We have surrendered and admitted our life has become unmanageable. I feel no peace, just incredible emptiness. It permeates my every thought.

I can't sleep. I can't eat, I can't think. I can't cry. I feel numb. Give me a bowl of ice cream. I need a nightly sugar fix.

I zip up the suitcases. My part of the plan is done until next weekend. The dreaded move-in day will be next Sunday. I carry the bags down the stairs, roll them to the closet under the stairway, push them in, and close the door.

I think about all the positive things about placing Mom in the Memory Care facility. She will be in a safe place; they will monitor her meds, bathe her daily, and keep her busy with activities. She won't be bored. She won't be angry at Dad. She won't walk out of the house unnoticed. The staff will be equipped to deal with her disease. Dad will be relieved. Dad won't have to fight with her daily. He won't have stress and anxiety on an hourly basis. He won't have to walk on eggshells. He can take care of himself. He can work uninterrupted. He can have his life back. I realize his list also applies to me, but it doesn't bring me peace. My stomach hurts. My heart aches.

The positive list is long. The negative list is short—I'm losing my mom, and my dad is losing his wife. Period. But haven't we already lost her? And haven't we lost ourselves?

Will our home still be a home without my mother? The nest of love and security she built unraveled one twig at a time. Our home will look the same, but it will be as empty as the little peek-a-boo birdhouse that sits outside on the carport.

It's time for Mom to fly away. My mom is leaving her nest, and we will never be the same.

CHAPTER FOURTEEN
THE LAST BEIGNET

"I'm going to meet Mom and Dad for dinner on Friday night," my sister Erin tells me over the phone. It's her last designated weekend with them. This is the last weekend before we move my mother into the Memory Care facility on Sunday.

"I want them to be with me on Friday night. I'm doing the *Meanwhile, Back at Cafe Du Monde...* show for the Louisiana Marathon kickoff. It will be the last time she sees the show, and she always enjoys it. Can you let me take them on Friday night?" I pleaded.

"Okay, then I will pick her up on Saturday morning and then have them over Saturday night for dinner," Erin replies.

258

I hang up my cell phone, and reality hits me. The plan is for Shannan and Rob to deliver Mom on Sunday morning to her new life in the Memory Care unit at an assisted living facility. On Saturday morning, we will move her things into her new room while she is with Erin. It makes me sick to think about it.

I have done everything to avoid thinking of this moment. Packing up Mom's things has been a mental distraction. I will not give up having her with me on Friday night for my show. Period. End of discussion.

Since I created the first *Meanwhile, Back at Cafe Du Monde...* show in 2010, my mom and Dad have been to every show I produced in Louisiana. She loves hearing life stories about food shared by local foodies and personalities.

The Louisiana Marathon kick-off show promises to be a lot of fun. We have a great group of people sharing their stories, including sponsors and marathoners, and it will end with a jazz band on stage. Mom will love it!

My parents are both fabulous storytellers! I inherited the storytelling gene from them. However, my need to perform probably began the day my dad received *The Music Man* album in the mail from his new record club. He played it on the stereo console, and I soon learned every song. At five years old, I would stand on the living room coffee table singing "Gary, Indiana" at the top of my lungs. With two little sisters by that time, it was my way of saying, "Look at me! Watch me shine!"

Soon, my mom enrolled me in dance class, and I loved every minute. I remember her making my costumes for my first dance review. It was a ballet hula dance, and I wore a pink hula outfit with a plastic lei. From the moment I stepped onto the stage in the spotlight, shaking my hips, I loved performing. At my yearly dance recitals, Mom was backstage doing my make-up and hair, dressing me in the sparkly costumes before sending me off with a big kiss and saying, "I'm so proud of you, Peggy!" She would scurry off to her seat in the front row, joining my dad, who captured it all with his movie camera.

After the recital, there were flowers, cards, and gifts, followed by a treat stop at Krispy Kreme for chocolate iced donuts or Shoney's Big Boy for chocolate cake layered with vanilla ice cream with chocolate sauce, whipped cream, and a cherry on top.

In 10th grade, I wore Mom's wedding "going away" wool suit with a matching hat to play a pushy stage mother in a play called *A Date with Judy*. My mother laughed hysterically watching my performance, and the audience followed. I was hooked on theatre, acting, and loved all my theatre buddies.

The years of drama class and dance recitals led to my earning a degree in Speech and Drama Education from Louisiana State University. After graduating, I followed a boyfriend to Houston, where I promptly qualified for my Screen Actors Guild card by getting cast in a commercial for a fried chicken chain. I was the girl behind the counter with a welcoming smile. "Welcome to Hartz," I said repeatedly to the camera.

Years of doing commercials, industrial films, and print work led me to New York City, where I struggled to find work in commercial and off-off-Broadway productions while working at law firms. When I was cast as a "Mom" in a Burger King commercial, my parents happened to be in New York visiting me and came to the set to watch me bite continuously into a Whopper with smiling eyes. They also laughed when they saw the bucket at my feet, where I'd spit after each bite. The reality behind the glamor!

It had been years since I auditioned for anything, as I had transitioned into meeting and event producing in Los Angeles, when I created my own show with *Meanwhile, Back at Cafe Du Monde...* after being inspired in 2009 by my friend Lisa's "Coconut Pie and a Bottle of Wine" story over Thanksgiving. The show has been produced across the country, featuring hundreds of people who share their life stories about food.

A Baton Rouge event producer who produces the Louisiana Marathon had seen the *Meanwhile, Back at Cafe Du Monde...* show the year before and asked me to produce it for the Marathon kickoff event.

On Friday, Mom, Dad, Jimmy, and I arrived early at the convention center, where a stage is set up on the edge of the marathon trade show. The convention center is buzzing with the marathoners registering for the big run the next morning.

Soon, I'm on stage checking the microphones with the stage crew after setting up a table on stage with the Café Du Monde mugs, napkin holder, and, of course, a plate of beignets. The little pillows of decadence, or fried donuts, that I speak of in my opening monologue are, unfortunately, not from Café Du Monde. I didn't have time to drive to New Orleans. These beignets are from the next best thing— Coffee Call in Baton Rouge.

"Can I have one?" Mom asks, standing at the edge of the stage, pointing at the beignets. She looks thin and a bit disheveled tonight, but I think she may grasp that I am setting up for the show. If you were to tell anyone that we are placing my mom in a Memory Care assisted living facility in two days for her Alzheimer's, they probably wouldn't believe it.

"Sure, Mom," I said, and I handed her a beignet wrapped in a napkin.

As I meet with the storytellers on stage, explaining the line-up, I look down and see my mom sitting there eating her beignet. She looks like a little child, smiling at everyone as powdered sugar lands on her lap. Dad leans over, brushes the sugar off her black pants, and she gives him a bite of her beignet.

I open the show with my food story and then introduce the other storytellers. Their stories are funny and touching. Mom loves every minute. She has always loved this show. She has loved anything that I did creatively. How will I continue to be creative without her love and support? I just don't know.

After the show, everyone mingles, while I sign *The Meanwhile, Back at Cafe Du Monde...* coffee table books for the audience members who purchase them from a local bookseller who has set up a table. I give the storytellers a signed book as a token of my appreciation. One of the storytellers, Uncle Larry, has his Louisiana "Stew in a Few" products for sale, and we purchased some to take home. His lovely Cajun wife and sister are there. They are fun-loving, gracious, and very sweet to us. They rave about the show, are proud of Larry, and ask me to sign the book for them. Mom loves meeting them. They ask her to sign one of her recipes featured in the book.

Troy Kleinpeter, my friend and photographer who has taken pictures of every show, is here tonight and snapped a few photos of my parents and me on the stage and a photo of Mom and me with the plate of beignets.

The convention center security is locking up for the night, and we are the last ones to leave. Jimmy has moved the car to the entrance, and we walk out the front door with Dad carrying my box of props.

"Y'all want to go get dinner?" I ask them.

"Sure. Where do you want to go?" Dad says.

"Let's check out White Star Market," I suggest.

We soon stand in the middle of the specialty food court market, glancing around at the food stall options. Dad and Mom decided to get pizza, while Jimmy and I ordered tacos. We meet at the community table in the middle of the room and share our food.

This is the last supper. A lifetime of going out to dinner with my parents, and this is how it ends with tacos and a pizza. It seems so uneventful.

Driving home, Mom and I are sitting in the back seat holding hands. My foot touches the white paper bag of leftover beignets from the show, and I reach down and pick up the bag.

"Do you want a beignet, Mom?"

"Sure!"

The beignets are crushed in the bag, damp from the humidity, and limp with the weight of the powdered sugar, but they are still good enough to eat. I never met a beignet I couldn't eat!

We sat in the back seat of the car, eating our beignets, getting powdered sugar all over ourselves and the car seat. This will be the last beignet I eat with my mom.

We devour the soggy beignets and then lick our fingers.

"Yummy!" I say.

"Lalicious," she says, and we giggle together.

My mom started saying "Lalicious" instead of "Delicious" a few years ago. It drives my sisters crazy. I think it is perfect, especially for these stale beignets. I want to hold on to every moment with her. Every "lalicious moment." I want to remember sitting in the back of our Toyota Corolla, eating our beignets and licking our fingers. I don't want to ever forget this night with my mother.

If life is delicious, the perfect word is lalicious. She pronounces it lalicious, as in Louisiana delicious. Life is short, and we need to remember how frickin delicious it is!

On Saturday morning, after Erin picks Mom up, Jimmy and I drive to the assisted living facility with our car loaded with Mom's clothes in secret suitcases and bags of framed pictures. A sweet older woman welcomes us at the front lobby. She explains the protocol. We are to sign in and out each time we visit. She gives us the room number and the secret code for the Memory Care unit. Rolling the suitcases down the hall, we passed through the dining area of the regular assisted living. A few older residents sit at their tables, talking as the workers clear away the breakfast dishes. I wish my mother could be in this section.

We punch in the secret code and walk down a long hall looking for her room number. We pass the Memory Care dining area and see a few residents asleep in their wheelchairs. Others are sitting in an alcove watching a woman lead them in a game. She throws the ball to them, and they catch it. Some laugh. Some just stare ahead.

A friendly caregiver sits at a table with older women, and they color in adult coloring books with colored markers. She plays oldies but goodies music from her phone, and she sings along. Mom will like her.

We pass a counter, and a woman standing behind it introduces herself to us and then points down the hall toward Mom's room. We find my brother-in-law and my nephew busy hanging large, framed artwork. Shannan and Rob delivered the furniture earlier this morning. My other brother-in-law arrives to set up Mom's television. Two days ago, we unhooked the small TV in the kitchen to bring it to her room. A maintenance man comes to hook up the cable. It is a group effort to make Mom's new space her home.

Jimmy and I unzip the suitcases and unpack her clothes, hanging shirts, pants, and jackets in the closet. I place her underwear and nightgowns in her dresser drawers. Jimmy sets the framed pictures on the dresser and end tables.

Kelly arrives with brand new, expensive-looking bedding, and we make the bed. The new bedding is a pretty dusty pink with matching pillow shams. She bought brand new sheets and towels in the same dusty pink color.

"Mom will love this. The chenille bedspread reminds me of the one Nanny used to have when we were kids," I tell Kelly.

"I know that's why I bought it," Kelly says. We barely look at each other as we are both ready to cry. It all seems unreal.

I placed the little red plastic bird that Mom and I bought at Dollar Tree a year ago on the windowsill. Soon, the sunlight activates the solar panel on the bird, and the wings begin to flap. This may bring her some comfort of familiarity. She loved this little bird. For the last few years, it has sat on the kitchen windowsill, wings fluttering in the sunlight.

I am feeling numb. I need a shot of the sun to make me feel alive. We are going through the motions, and nobody discusses what's really happening here. We are preparing Mom for her new life of being caged in. She will never flap her wings again. There will be no sunlight to activate her spirit.

The room is complete. It looks lovely. I often think about how Mom repeatedly told Dad she wanted to move away and get her own apartment. Will she like having this studio apartment, or will it be a prison cell? Will her mind even know the difference?

"Thank you in advance for taking care of my mother," I tell each caregiver. They smile and try to make us feel comfortable in our awkwardness.

The woman at the front desk gives us each a key to Mom's room as we sign out. She notices my tears. "It is going to be okay. I know it's hard, but we will take good care of her. It's best if you all stay away for a couple of weeks so she has time to adjust."

I nod my head, but I can't answer, or I will start crying. The lump in my throat is huge. Jimmy and I walked to the car, and he put the key to Mom's room on our keyring.

"Do you want to grab lunch?" he asks.

I lean my head against the window and sob, so he just starts the car and drives home. I walked straight up to bed for a nap and slept all afternoon, waking up right when Mom and Dad were leaving to go to Erin's for dinner.

270

Our Saturday "date night" consisted of me lying on the sofa downstairs watching my TV shows while Jimmy was upstairs watching his. I found leftovers in the fridge to zap in the microwave. We each took our trays of food to our TVs. We didn't talk about it because we knew I would cry.

On Sunday morning, we act like it is just a regular Sunday. Mom and Dad were already awake, drinking coffee in the living room when I came down in my robe. I grabbed my coffee and walked around the room, opening the blinds. We need sunshine on this heartbreaking day. I joined my mother on our old green sofa. I turned the TV on, and we mindlessly watched it. After I finished my coffee, I lay my head on her lap. I knew Shannan and Rob would walk in to take her away any moment.

She strokes my hair. We don't talk. I hear their car pull into the driveway, and moments later, as the back door opens, I spring up.

Shannan and Rob walked into the house and entered the living room.

"You ready, Mom? Let's go get some breakfast," Shannan tells her.

"OK," she says while Shannan grabs her hands and pulls her up from the sofa.

"See you later, Dad," Shannan says. He is sitting stoically in his chair.

And just like that, my mother is gone.

"I think I am going to blow leaves from the deck," Dad tells me, getting up and walking out of the house.

I lie down on the sofa and roll over, so my face is in the old green pillows. I cry my heart out. Soon, the leaf blower is drowning out my sobs.

An hour later, the phone rang. I pick it up in the living room, and Dad picks it up from the kitchen.

"Well, it's done. I just did the one thing Mom told me would be the worst thing we could ever do to her." Shannan says through her tears.

"I'm so sorry. Thank you," I said.

The welcoming committee of two friendly caregivers met my mom and escorted her to her room, with Shannan and Rob following behind them. They distracted her by chit-chatting about everything and nothing. Once in her room, Shannan, my strong sister, stepped forward to drop the bomb. Mom was on one side of the bed, and Shannan was on the other.

"Mom, look at me. Do you know how worried you have been about your memory? Well, this is a great place to help you with it. You trust me, right, Mom? You need to trust me."

"Is this forever?" Mom asked.

"No, it's just for now," Shannan told her, and Mom believed her.

We all want to believe Shannan—that this is only temporary. Dad, my sisters, Shannan, and I cling to the hope that, by some miracle, our mother will get well. We want to believe she will come home again.

Mom's Easy Campground Beignets

Ingredients:

Two (or more) cans of refrigerator biscuits (you can never have enough)
4 cups of vegetable oil
1 box of powdered sugar

Instructions:

Open the cans of biscuits and cut each biscuit in half.
Heat the cooking oil in a Dutch oven or deep-frying pan over medium-high heat.
Test the temperature by placing a small piece of dough in the oil. If it starts bubbling around the beignet, it is hot enough.
Drop cut biscuits into hot oil in a single layer. Do not overcrowd.
Using a slotted spoon, turn the donuts once they are golden brown on the bottom.
When donuts are golden brown on each side, remove them with slotted spoon and drain them on a plate covered with paper towels.
Continue with the remaining biscuits until they are done and drained.
Pour powdered sugar into a large bowl.
Toss the beignets around until they are covered with powdered sugar.

Yield:

Serves 8 (but it will never be enough!)

Family Notes:

Growing up, my mother would make these simple beignets when camping in our pop-up camper. My dad would set up a Coleman stove outside on a picnic table. We would help my mother cut the canned biscuits and then take turns shaking a paper bag with the beignets and the powdered sugar. The delicious smell of beignets frying would bring neighboring campers to our site. Nothing is more appetizing than a hot beignet covered with powdered sugar and dipped in hot chocolate or coffee. It is heaven!

If you don't have the time to make beignets from scratch or use the Café Du Monde beignet mix, which I hear is not too difficult, this is the easier, softer way to make little pillows of decadence, as I call them!

CHAPTER FIFTEEN
THE BABY DOLLS

Mom has been gone for two days. It's hard to believe she isn't coming home. Dad and I walk around in a stupor. The house seems so quiet and empty—empty as our hearts. The Memory Care supervisor advised us to stay away for two weeks so that Mom can adjust to her new routine and home. They told us we could call anytime. Each day, we take turns calling.

"Your mom is doing great," they tell us.

"Were you able to get her in the shower?"

"Yes."

"Is she eating?"

"Yes."

"Can we come see her tomorrow?"

"No, she needs a few more days to get adjusted," they tell us.

"This is so hard," I tell the caregiver, choking back tears.

"I know it is, but this is the best way!"

It's the same message each day—she is doing well, eating, taking showers, and has made friends.

The wait to see her is excruciating. Is she happy there? Is she angry with us? How can we stay away? We are going crazy with the wait.

Life moves forward. I go to work. I cook dinner. I clean. I wash clothes—including her last dirty ones I find in the hamper. After dinner, I sit on the old green sofa and watch television. It's just not the same without her on the other end.

Dad sits across the room, reading. Jimmy is upstairs in his den watching his TV. This is our new norm. It's quiet. It's peaceful. Everyone is in their own space. We no longer have to struggle with Mom. I'm missing the struggle. I'm missing my mom.

"Do you think I can take your mother out of Memory Care on Thursday night and take her to see *Jersey Boys*? We bought tickets a few months ago with the Fairwood group," Dad mentioned at dinner the day after we moved Mom.

The Fairwood group has been friends for over fifty years. They all belonged to the Fairwood Country Club, where they played tennis and golf. The club is long gone, but their friendship survived.

"No, Dad, you can't do that."

"She was looking forward to it. It's one of her favorite Broadway shows," he says.

"Let me see what my sisters think. I'll text them," I tell him, though I already know.

"*No, he can't do that*," Shannan texts.

"*Not a good idea,*" Kelly texts.

"*He'll never be able to get her to return to Memory Care if he takes her out,*" Shannan adds.

"I guess I will just give the tickets away," Dad says, looking sad and lost.

"Dad, I will go with you," I tell him.

"OK," he says listlessly.

My parents have seen *The Jersey Boys* several times—in New York, in New Orleans—and we all watched the movie together. Mom loves all the Frankie Valli songs. She would have loved to see it again with all of her friends. This sucks.

"Do you want to go get something to eat before the play?" I ask him,

"No, we can just eat at home before we go downtown."

I understand. My dad doesn't know how to live life without my mom. None of us knows how to live life without Mom. The void is real and cruel. He feels like a widower, but his wife hasn't died. She slowly disappeared, becoming a woman, he no longer recognized. She's now across town, and he can't even visit her until Memory Care gives us the green light.

On Thursday evening, we drove downtown. As we walk into the theatre, the Fairwood friends light up when they see us. I love this group!

"How are you, Myles?" they ask Dad with eyes full of love and concern. They know Mom has been moved to Memory Care. They can't imagine what we are going through. A few of the women are teary-eyed.

"I'm glad you came with your dad," they tell me. I need their hugs. They all stand and hug us as we slide through the row to our seats. This play will be a good distraction, I think—a few hours' escape.

It works until the Jersey Boys sing "Sherry." I grab Dad's hand, and I start to cry. This is Mom's song! The words, *"Sherry, can you come out tonight?"* hit hard. My Mom can't "come out" anymore. I'm sitting in her seat at one of her favorite plays. I just know all her friends are thinking the same thing. Sherry baby, we miss you! It's just not the same without you, Mom.

We managed to enjoy the show as much as possible. It's hard not to enjoy *The Jersey Boys*, but sadness colors everything. Seeing the Fairwood friends is a shot in the arm. They all love Mom and ask us to let them know when they can visit her as we say our goodbyes in the lobby.

"Your mom would have loved this," Dad says as we pull out of the parking lot.

"I know, Dad. Let's get her an Alexa device for her room and set up a Frankie Valli Pandora station."

"That's a great idea. I will go buy one tomorrow."

On Sunday, Dad decides he is going to visit Mom. He doesn't care that it has only been one week. He needs to see her. The guilt and grief tear him up.

"I want to bring the Alexa. I want her to listen to her favorite music," he says, and off he goes.

He arrives at lunchtime. He sits at the table with Mom, and they even bring him a plate. She gives him the cold shoulder at first, then warms up. After lunch, they watch a movie with the group. She reaches over and holds his hand. The caregivers are friendly and attentive. He walks her back to her room, and she falls asleep on her bed. He reads for a while, then quietly slips out of the room. Before leaving, he checks in with the supervisor, who says that in the first few days, Mom was furious. She paced the hallway and convinced someone walking out of the unit that she was just visiting. They let her out, and the front receptionist noticed her walking toward the main entrance door and stopped her. She was livid at us for placing her here and angry with the staff.

"She's doing much better now," the supervisor says.

"I think we did the right thing," Dad tells me, but I can see he doesn't quite believe it yet.

"Can I go see her?" I ask him.

"I think so. Ask your sisters."

They don't want us to overwhelm her, so only one sister at a time! Shannan texts. We coordinate days.

I'm scared the first time I visit, but I'm fine once I see her smile, feel her hug, and sit holding her hand. I joined the activities. We colored. I do most of the talking, but that is nothing new. Mom hadn't been talkative in a while.

Dad goes to visit every day. Soon, my sisters stopped coordinating; we just go when we can and bump into each other. One sister arrives as the other one leaves. Sometimes we're there at the same time, and Mom likes the commotion. We sit in her room. We eat her snacks. We tell stories. We pull out the photo albums and flip through them. We play Barbra Streisand, Celine Dion, and Frankie Valli on her Alexa. For a few minutes, we forget we are not at home.

One afternoon, a one-man band performs, and I sit with Mom. Soon, I pull her up, and we dance. We laugh. She smiles at her new friends, and the caregivers seem to love her. I'm not surprised. Everyone always loved my mom. She was always the light in the room. She always made everyone feel special.

One afternoon, family friends visited her, and as they walked through the assisted living area to reach Memory

Care, they saw a band playing and people dancing. It looked fun, so when they found her sitting in her room alone, staring at the TV, they decided they should take her to hear the music. They didn't know the protocol and just walked her out. By the second song, Mom was up dancing with one of the workers.

When they went to leave, she told them, "Go ahead. I'm going to stay." They left her smiling, clapping, and singing along, unaware that she had no idea how to return to Memory Care. The staff found her wandering around the halls and immediately called Dad, instructing him to please tell his friends they must sign her out and in from the Memory Care desk and deliver her back to her room. When he told me, I had to laugh. It tickled me—it was exactly like something Mom would do. She may have Alzheimer's, but her spirit isn't broken. She was still enjoying the party. She's still making new friends!

Dad called our friends; they were horrified and felt awful. I took the phone. They had no idea how far my mom's disease had progressed. I reassured them.

"It's okay. Honestly, we needed a laugh. I haven't laughed in several months."

It's been over three months since we moved Mom, I think, as I pulled into the driveway to visit her. I sit in the car for a few minutes, checking my phone for texts, calls, Facebook, Instagram—anything to avoid going inside.

It's still hard to believe Mom lives here. It seems like we have failed her. I failed her. I know she is getting better care, but the reality that my mother is never coming home is hard to swallow. They say it takes ninety days for a new habit to get easier. This isn't getting easier; it's getting harder. Each time I see her, her eyes are more distant, her body frailer. She barely smiles. She hardly speaks.

As I walk the path from the parking lot to the entrance, I wonder what is more painful: coming home to find her arguing with Dad pre-Memory Care or seeing her here among Alzheimer's patients who are further along. Everywhere you look, it's a reminder of what's going to come.

I sign in at the front desk. The receptionist is young, perky, and always greets me with a smile. To the right of the reception desk is the "lounge," where some assisted living residents sit and play cards, laughing over their iced tea and snacks provided at the bar. I wish my mom were one of them. Some evenings there's a happy hour with wine or beer; the lounge is packed. Dad occasionally brings Mom to the activity room when there's live music. She enjoyed it. Music always makes Mom come alive.

I walk up the stairs to the Memory Care door and check my phone for the security code. It changes every few weeks.

I punch in the secret code, and the door opens automatically, then shuts quickly. If you hold it open, a loud alarm blares. I know because I've set it off, and staff come running to ensure no one escapes. This is a locked unit. When Mom stepped through these doors, she lost any independence she had left.

We no longer visit daily. Staff told us that every time we left, she became agitated, and it took a day or two to get her back to her "new norm," whatever that is. Dad has cut down on his visits to every other day.

Today, I found my mom sitting with one of her Alzheimer's patient friends in the living room. They're both holding baby dolls. Miss Alma is a sweet woman who usually has both baby dolls in her arms. She carries them everywhere.

In the corner is a baby bed with baskets of doll clothes. The staff told us that Alzheimer's patients often love dolls—they're comforting.

Mom looks up and sees me. Her face lights up, and she says, "There's my girl!"

Today she doesn't remember my name, but I'm okay with being "her girl." I sit beside her, and she shows me her baby.

"Isn't she precious?" she gushes.

"She's adorable, Mom. Can I hold the baby?"

"Sure," she replies, handing over the doll.

We watch the news, and I make small talk.

"Where's Dad been? He hasn't come to visit me in ages," she asks.

"He's busy working," I say, although I know that he was here for lunch.

A caregiver comes to take them to dinner. I walk Mom into the dining room and sit with her. She taps the top of her lips with her fingers. She's done this for years; I know now it helps her anxiety. It's one of those weird quirks that drove all of us crazy, especially my dad. Being hard of hearing, he found it difficult to understand her when she was speaking with her hands over her mouth. He'd ask her to stop. She'd get upset and embarrassed. It breaks my heart thinking about it now, but Dad was doing the best he could.

The attendant sets a plate of roast beef, mashed potatoes, and peas in front of Mom. She just stares at the food. I handed her the fork.

"That looks delicious, Mom!" I say, encouraging her to eat a few bites. She then pushes the plate away and tries the banana pudding, shakes her head, and pushes it away, too. Dinner is over.

Frustrated, I took a few bites. It's pretty good. I'd finish it as I'm hungry, but I'm embarrassed to eat my mother's food.

Miss Kathleen, a tiny Irishwoman, sits across the table from us. "I need a glass of milk. If I could just get a nice glass of milk, then I could go to bed," she says over and over. The caregiver tells her she can't have milk because of her medicine, and she drops her head into her hands and starts to cry. It is heartbreaking.

Just give her a fricken glass of milk. I can't bear to watch.

"Mom, ready to go to your room?" I asked standing.

"Yes."

I help her stand, and as we walk away, she says, "Why won't they let her have any milk?"

"I don't know, Mom."

We walked down the hall. I turned on the TV. She lies down on the bed. I noticed her plants need watering, and I jumped up to water them. I look in her closet and organize her clothes. One of her shoes is missing. A sweater is in the dirty clothes hamper. I take it out. It needs to be hand-washed. I'll take it home and clean it. I probably shouldn't have brought this sweater, but I wanted to bring her things that make her happy. Another level of denial peels away. Mom needs pull-up pants, long-sleeved cotton shirts, and slip-on shoes, the essentials. She doesn't need dry-clean-only sweaters.

Crystal, the kind nurse with the beautiful smile, our medicine fairy, comes in with Mom's meds.

"What's this for?" Mom asks.

"It's your medicine, Mom."

"Oh, okay," and she swallows. It's easier here. At home, meds were a daily ordeal. Exhausting. What's their magic? Crystal says some days are better than others.

Sometimes she crushes the pills and stirs them into a little cup of pudding.

The caregiver comes in to help Mom into her nightgown and get her ready for bed. I know I'm just in the way now—my cue to leave.

"Love you, Mom. Goodnight. I'll see you tomorrow." I kiss her, knowing I won't be here tomorrow. It's too painful. It's too sad. My daily visits have dwindled to twice a week.

"Bye," she says to me. I'm amazed at how my mom has accepted this as her home. She has never asked me to take her back. I'm relieved—I wouldn't know how to deal with it—but saddened. Doesn't she want to come home?

It's 6:00 p.m., and the residents are being tucked in like little children. I punch the code, slip out, head down the stairs, and walk the path to the lot. I put one foot in front of the other. Get to the car before I cry.

I pass a woman about my age, on her way in. We share a knowing smile. We are members of a club of daughters losing our mothers daily to the Big A.

We need to get my mom a baby doll. Shannan mentioned it last month, but none of us has bought one. I'd feel much better knowing she has something to hug when she sleeps.

The following week, my Aunt Margaret and her daughter, Cindy, visited with gifts: twin baby dolls, a boy and a girl, with cute outfits and blankets. Mom loves them. The next time I visit, she can't wait to show off her adored babies. We sit side by side, each holding a doll. She talks to them sweetly, takes the hat off, and puts it back on. We agree they're precious. She smiles at them. I love seeing her happy.

My mom isn't talking much, but with the baby dolls, she comes alive and carries on coherent conversations. The baby dolls are a lifeline.

When my mom was a little girl, her mother would take the bus on Sunday mornings to borrow a baby from a New Orleans orphanage for the day. She'd bring the baby home, they'd play all day, and return the baby in the evening. My mom adored these babies. If they didn't like their names, they'd rename them for the day. One baby had a very old-fashioned name, like Hazel or Josephine, and they called her Peggy. She was a favorite. When I was born, Mom named me Peggy. I was her first real baby doll—her first child—born thirteen months after my parents got married. She cried every month when she wasn't pregnant. She couldn't wait to have a baby.

My mom is a baby whisperer. She loves babies—her babies, her grandbabies, her friends' babies, and her friends' grandbabies—any baby. She loves to talk about babies. She loves to look at baby pictures.

I keep thinking about the day my niece, Mackenzie, told us she was pregnant last summer. The whole family met for Sunday brunch at a favorite Mexican restaurant. Mackenzie wanted Mom next to her. She and her husband, Eric, made the big announcement with the sonogram. Mom's face lit up like a Christmas tree. She cried happy tears—her first great-grandchild. The baby is due in April—a boy they'll call Tripp! I hope Mom gets to meet him.

Mom is tired and lies down. I lie down beside her, and we each cuddled a baby doll. I ask Alexa to play relaxing piano music. Soon, Mom is fast asleep. I slip out of bed, placing my baby doll next to hers. I lean over and kissed her.

"I love you, Mom! Goodnight. Sleep tight. Don't let the bedbugs bite."

As I closed the door, I remembered my mother tucking me in as a child and saying those exact words. I want to stay and hold her all night. Instead, I'm going home—to her home. A home that was once filled with a rich, beautiful life.

I long for the days when I would come back to visit my family in Baton Rouge and Mom would cook my favorite meals. My sisters would come over with the kids, and they would pull out the toys from the closet under the stairs. The house was loud with laughter, kids shrieking, and the brothers-in-law goofing on us. I miss those days. I miss the sounds of life in a place now quiet and empty.

My mom's spirit was fierce. Her love for her family was unending—sometimes overwhelming—but constant and unconditional. I look back now and realize how much I took it for granted. I'd have a hard day with her right now just to have her home.

Arriving home, I walk into the house and go straight into her closet. I pulled out her old red robe, still hanging in her closet. After showering, I put on her robe. It still smells like her favorite perfume - Estee Lauder *Pleasures*. It reminds me of Mom before Alzheimer's, dressed up and ready to go out on the town.

The simple pleasures of my mother in her better days are everywhere. I will continue to look for them and cherish the memories. Still, right now, I'm okay, lying on the old green sofa with her red robe embracing me, watching our show—*Dancing with the Stars*—and knowing she is still alive across town, holding her precious baby dolls.

CHAPTER SIXTEEN
HOSPITAL MADNESS

I find my mom sitting at a table in the middle of the kitchen area of the dining room, where they serve the food for the Memory Care residents at assigned dining room tables. My mom doesn't have a specific seat. I find her in different spots whenever I visit, and I have no idea why. She stopped eating a few weeks ago, so they are "watching" her—which means she sits at a table in the kitchen, and the servers scurry around her, giving her extra attention for her food issues.

A plate of chicken, rice, and green beans sits in front of her. I know she can't possibly eat this food. She has lost her top dental bridge and can no longer put her bottom bridge in her mouth. How can she chew with only a few front top and bottom teeth?

"She doesn't look pretty anymore without her teeth. I want to take her to the dentist to get another top bridge made and get the dental assistant to teach her how to put her bottom teeth in," Dad told me last month.

"That's crazy, Dad. She will just lose the bridge again. It's not worth the $2,500 to get another bridge made." I told him.

Dad sighed and shook his head sadly. I don't know what is more heartbreaking: Mom without teeth or Dad pleading his case. My sisters tell him the same thing:

"Don't waste your money, Dad. She will just lose the bridge again," Shannan says.

"It's not a good idea to take her out of the Memory Care," Kelly adds.

I lean down and hug Mom. She just looks at me. I don't think she knows who I am today. I hate it.

I walk down the hall to her room to get a protein drink from her refrigerator. Dad stocked the fridge with yogurts, protein drinks, Jell-O, soda, bottled water, and juice boxes. Kelly filled the cabinet with a family-size carton of Goldfish and individually wrapped cookie snacks. I brought some of her favorite candy and mints. Everything is untouched. Mom doesn't eat or drink these things because she doesn't remember they are here. I'm sure she doesn't even know what a refrigerator is anymore. She only eats snacks when we're here to hand them to her.

Sometimes, I stuff my face with the Goldfish because I'm usually here at dinnertime. Pepperidge Farm Goldfish are addictive—you can't eat just a handful. It's handful after handful. Mindless eating, or nervous eating, is my crutch when I visit Mom. I could request a plate or eat her untouched dinner, but it never feels right.

I grab a small peach yogurt, a chocolate protein drink, and a cranberry juice box, then lock her door so the other patients don't intrude. We have learned the rules: **Lock the door.** It's probably why her clothes, robe, favorite pink blanket, and some of her shoes have gone missing, even though we have stamped her name on everything with the two "Sherry Sweeney" stamps Kelly ordered.

The staff told us that Mom once wandered into another room and climbed into someone else's bed. They found her sleeping. She wasn't happy when they woke her to move.

"She was so angry at us," they said. *Lock the Door* is forever imprinted on my brain.

I hustle back down the hall and sit with her at the table. A caregiver hands me a straw, and I hold the protein

296

drink to Mom's mouth. She takes a few sips, then shakes her head. I distract her with conversation and try to spoon in a bite of yogurt.

"It's peach, Mom. You love peach yogurt," I say. She takes two bites—end of story.

I hold the juice carton to her lips, and she tries to sip but doesn't suck long enough.

"Suck harder, Mom." She tries again and gets a few drops. I keep trying, but this is probably the best we'll manage today. Pathetic. I feel defeated.

Mom is wasting away right before our eyes. When she moved into Memory Care, she was a size 14. Now her 12s hang on her, so she is a size 10 or an 8. She has lost 20 in four months. Maybe I should move in here. I need to lose 20 pounds.

"Peggy, please go shopping with Dad to get Mom some new clothes. All of her clothes are hanging on her. Her pants were falling off her today," Shannan tells me.

So I went to the local Goodwill, picked up more petite pull-up elastic pants, cotton shirts, and nightgowns. I took them home, washed them, and packed them in a rolling suitcase.

I'm amazed they get Mom to wear pajamas—it's a strict rule here.

"All residents must have nightclothes on, or we get written up by the morning caregivers," an evening attendant, Tiffany, explained. I can only imagine the arguing they endure with Mom, but maybe they've just got the magic touch.

The caregivers at this Memory Care are lovely. They all stop by the table in the kitchen and give Mom a little love. "Sherry Berry," they exclaim, hugging her and making small talk with her. She smiles back. She loves the attention. She loves to be called Sherry Berry.

"Do you want to watch the news, Mom?" I say.

"We are getting ready to have Christian devotion in the living room," Deana announces enthusiastically.

Deana is a beautiful, warm, and vibrant woman—full makeup, fake eyelashes, and long acrylic nails. I love her energy. She's attentive to Mom. I can't imagine spending the time getting dolled up to work here. I can barely manage to wash my hair twice a week, and I only wear makeup when I'm going out in public. Dry shampoo is my best friend.

"Sounds great, Deana. I could use some devotion." I say. She hugs Mom and me, and I walk Mom into the living room. We find two chairs along the wall as the caregivers wheel in the residents. Many of them are in wheelchairs. Some seem totally out of it, others are alert, and some babble non-stop—but nothing makes sense.

There is one woman, possibly in her 50s, who curses and screams constantly. Maybe her dementia comes out like Tourette's. They eventually walk her to her room, and she curses all the way down the hall. Other times, she sits in her room with the door open wide, singing the same verse of a song repeatedly. It's maddening.

"She's awful," Mom exclaims. It is the first thing she has said to me all evening.

Deana reads from a Christian prayer book, shares a message of hope, then leads everyone in a prayer. She ends the 15-minute devotion by singing *Amazing Grace*. Mom and I joined in. It's unbelievable—she can barely talk anymore, yet she remembers every word of the first verse of Amazing Grace. It's AMAZING! A ray of hope in this grim situation. I am blessed at this moment.

By 6:30, the caregivers begin leading the residents to their rooms. Tiffany, one of my mom's favorites, helps her stand and takes her by the hand like a child. I hug and kiss her goodbye.

"I love you, Mom," I say.

She surprises me with, "Love you too!"

I stand watching them stroll down the hall before I turn and leave Memory Care.

Out in the car, I blasted the radio and pounded the steering wheel. "I hate you, Alzheimer's. It's not fair. I want my mom back!" I yell until my throat aches. An elderly gentleman standing in front of my car looks concerned. "I'm okay," I mouth. He nods, knowingly smiles, and continues towards the entrance, probably to see his wife.

I'm not okay. I feel like I'm going insane.

I text my sisters:

We need to tag team to see Mom every day. Make sure she has some protein drink, yogurt, and juice. She is wasting away. Weak. Barely spoke tonight.

Okay. Thanks for letting us know. Erin texts.

Thanks for going, Peg. Shannan texts.

I'll be there tomorrow. Kelly texts.

I drove home. I'm not crying tonight, I'm pissed. Angry at the world. Alzheimer's is a cruel way to die, a brutal way to lose my mother. I hate my life.

When I walk into the house, Jimmy comes down the stairs. He can tell by the look on my face that it has been a rough night. He hugs me and says, "22 seconds."

"Yes," I croak, and the tears finally fall. We read that a 22-second hug releases serotonin and drops you from your head to your heart. It does work sometimes, but I'm not in the mood tonight. He's holding me extra tight and counting, but I pull away at 12 seconds, resisting comfort. Sometimes you just need to wallow!

"That wasn't 22 seconds," he says.

"I'm hungry. I need to eat. Let me find something for dinner."

Dad walks into the kitchen from the living room,

"How was your mom?" he asks. I filled him in and tell him she barely ate again.

"I'll pick up some more protein drinks and yogurts at the store tomorrow," he says.

"Peach is her favorite," I suggest.

Does it matter? Peach, Coconut, Strawberry, whatever.

"What does it matter if she eats or not? She is not going to get any better." Jimmy lectures. He watched his father waste away in a New York nursing home for over three years." Dad and I just ignored him.

I pull out two cans of white albacore tuna fish and mix in some mayo, spicy mustard, celery, and relish in a plastic bowl. We sat at the table eating tuna sandwiches on toasted English Muffins. We barely talk. We just sit there chewing our food. We have no energy for chit-chat.

"Did you go see Mom today?" I ask Dad to break the silence.

"No, but I'll go tomorrow," Dad replies.

He is exhausted from the grind and can't make her eat. He told me she turns her head when he kisses her and tells him she hates him.

"You put me here!" she told him a few weeks ago.

He feels ashamed and sad. He sits by her side and tries to have a conversation. He tells her what he has been doing, what the girls are doing, what the grandkids are doing, and whatever he can think to say to fill the space.

How much can a spouse take? My sisters and I are all worried about Dad's health. He needs knee surgery on his left knee in the worst way. He hobbles these days but refuses to use a cane. The long walk from the parking lot to the front door of Memory Care and down the long halls is grueling for him.

"Do you want to watch Netflix?" I ask my dad after dinner. Jimmy heads to his upstairs man cave to watch his *CSI* reruns, his sports, or another round of *The Godfather* or *Goodfellas.* Dad and I settle into our routine. We sit and watch TV together. He pushes his big chair closer to the television while I curl up on the old green sofa. As one show ends and another begins, I hit pause on the program and go to the kitchen to get us water, hot tea, cookies, cake, or candy. Sometimes he requests another glass of wine or gets up to make himself whiskey on the rocks. We watch the shows with subtitles—his hearing aids never quite do the trick.

Streaming TV is our therapy. For a few hours, it wipes the slate clean—sadness, confusion, anger, regrets, dread. It numbs the grief of Mom and the Big A.

At 10:00 p.m., when we turn off the TV and head to bed, it all downloads back into my fried brain. Sleeping is impossible.

At the bottom of the stairs, I hug Dad goodnight.

"Thanks for dinner. That was great," he says, and I head upstairs. Dad always thanks me for fixing dinner, even if it's just a bowl of canned soup or a tuna sandwich.

I cook several times a week, always preparing enough for leftovers. Sometimes I make breakfast for dinner: eggs, sausage, biscuits, or English Muffins. Dad and I laugh, remembering how I would pitch a fit if Mom dared to make breakfast for dinner.

"Breakfast for dinner? That's gross!" I would say, as I stormed around the house like a teenage drama queen. Spoiled and ungrateful. How did they put up with me? Jimmy shakes his head when he hears this story.

"I loved it when my mom made breakfast for dinner!" he says.

"Shut up!" I snap.

"Forget about it," he grins, and we laugh.

Later that week, I found Mom in the small sitting room area outside her room. She is sitting there staring into space, tapping her fingers above her mouth.

"Mom?"

She just looks at me. It's heartbreaking. I get yogurt from the refrigerator and try to feed her a few bites. She looks horrible—pale and weak. I get bottled water, pour some in a cup, grab a straw, and bring it to her. She takes a few sips from the straw.

"Do you want to go lie down?" I ask her. She won't respond. I help her stand and walk her slowly to the room. At the bedside, I back her up and sit her on the bed. She collapses like a rag doll, eyes rolling back. OMG! I ran down the hall and find nurse Crystal at her cart dispensing meds to the residents.

"Something is wrong with my mom! Can you please check my mom's blood pressure?" I shout. She grabs her blood pressure cuff and follows me. Mom is lying there, just staring at the ceiling. Crystal takes her blood pressure and says, "Let me recheck it," and then calmly, "I think you need to take her to the emergency room. It's way too low."

Text flurry:

Mom's not doing well. Out of it and low blood pressure. Taking her to the hospital.

Scott and I will come to pick you and Mom up. We are on the way. Meet us at the front door! Erin texts.

I ran down the hall to grab a wheelchair, and one of the attendees came to help me lift her into the chair. It's not an easy task, as she is a dead weight. She has no color now, and I feel like she is dying.

Dad and the other sisters text back:

Take her to the Emergency Room at The General.

We will meet you there.

I wheel her down the hall, into the elevator, and out of the entrance. Erin and Scott are already there and helped get Mom into the car. I jump into my car and follow them. The hospital is only a few miles away.

Within minutes, we arrived at the Emergency Room and were escorted right in, thanks to my sister, Kelly, who is part of the hospital system and had called ahead.

Only one of us is allowed to go back with Mom at a time, so we take turns going in and out. It's crowded, and there are no rooms available. Mom is in the hallway on a gurney. They take blood for tests and put an IV into her arm to get fluids started. She is dehydrated, agitated, and confused. I'm with her when they wheel her down the hall for a chest X-ray and ultrasound.

Two nurses arrive, and one tells me, "We need a urine specimen from your mother."

"Good luck with that," I quip. I can't imagine trying to get Mom to pee in a cup. They roll their eyes at each other and take her into a room to insert a catheter to get the urine specimen. I can't watch it. It hurts me to even think about it, and Mom screams with agony. I held her hand.

"It's going to be okay, Mom."

Her urine is dark brown. Clearly, a bad UTI, which I learn is common for Alzheimer's patients because they have bad toileting habits. UTIs cause bacteria to enter the bloodstream, leading to disorientation, weakness, and potentially erratic behavior. UTIs are poisonous to the brain for older people.

At 11:00 p.m., she's still in the hallway waiting for a room. Shannan volunteers to stay for the night with her and sends us home. Mom hasn't moved into a hospital room until 1:30 a.m. It's a nightmare. Shannan is up all night with her. She keeps trying to get out of bed and picks at her IV.

I barely slept. When I woke up, Dad had already left for the hospital. I dressed quickly and grabbed some fresh clothes for Mom—pants, shirt, and a cute cardigan sweater for when she leaves. I hadn't packed this outfit when we moved Mom; I thought it was too fancy for Memory Care. Maybe it will make her feel better today.

I headed out the door at 7:30 a.m., stopping at McDonald's for Egg McMuffins and a giant coffee to drink in the car.

When I walked into the hospital room, Mom looked 75% better. She was sitting up and talking to Dad. I kissed her.

"I brought Egg McMuffins," I announced.

"I ate your mom's breakfast. She only had a bite of the grits," Dad says.

"I went down to the cafeteria for breakfast when Dad arrived," Shannan added.

"I'm on a diet," Erin chirped up from behind her iPad.

Kelly texted us she was on her way. "The Geriatrician wants to speak to us at 9:00," she added. I wonder what that means as I sit eating my cold Egg McMuffin.

At 8:30, Kelly, Jimmy, and Erin's husband, Scott, arrived. Then the Catholic priest walked in to give Mom the last rites. WHAT? Who requested this?

We look at each other anxiously, but we all gathered around Mom's bed to pray the *Our Father* with the priest. Mom smiled at him, took communion, and had no clue what was happening. We have no idea what this all means. All of the sisters are crying. Dad looks stunned.

What is this? Is she dying now— from Alzheimer's, starvation, or a Urinary Tract Infection? Holy Moly!

We are all in a daze. Jimmy and Scott joke around with Mom, and she laughs as we wait for the meeting with the doctor.

At 9:00, the doctor arrives with a team of four, including a hospice care representative. They pulled us into an empty room down the hall. Jimmy and Scott stayed back with Mom.

The conversation was a blur.

"She is not ready for hospice, but it could be soon," the doctor reports.

How soon?" Shannan asked.

"It could be weeks or months. We never know. Don't force your mother to eat. She could choke and then get pneumonia. Offer food, but don't push it. We will keep her here for another day for the UTI and continue treating her with antibiotics."

He suggested palliative care, the step before hospice. They will visit once or twice a week to help her bathe and perform exercises to keep her muscles moving. The hospice representative gives us a packet of information and explains that once we place Mom on hospice care, she won't be admitted to the hospital anymore, only comfort care. If she should get another UTI or anything else, she would just be given drugs to keep her comfortable.

The doctor was kind and informative, and the hospice rep was compassionate. My sister Kelly knows the doctor and tells us he is the best.

We walked out of the room, stunned. It's happening too fast. Mom has only been in Memory Care for four and a half months.

"Sherry, leave the IV alone," Jimmy tells Mom as we enter her room. She was picking at it again. She didn't ask where we'd been. Thank God! She is oblivious.

310

One by one, everyone left for work. Dad decided he needed a haircut and called his barber to see if he could get an appointment. I guess it is his way of checking out, and I don't blame him. You just found out your wife is nearing the end. What else can you do?

I stayed with Mom. She sat upright in the bed, and I climbed in next to her. We watched TV as she picked at the medical tape holding her IV.

"Mom, don't do that, or the needle will come out. You need the fluids."

"Why?"

"To make you feel better."

"I feel fine. I need to go to the bathroom."

"OK, I'll help you."

I unplug the IV from the wall unit and walk with her, dragging the IV pole behind us. I notice that she has an adult diaper under the hospital gown in the bathroom. She pulls it down and sits on the toilet. I stand there while she does her business, and when she finishes, she begins to wipe herself from back to front, which is why she has a UTI.

"Mom, let me help you."

"What are you doing? I can do it. Do you get your kicks out of this? GET OUT OF HERE," she yells at me.

"Fine! I don't know why you won't let me help you. I'm leaving."

I left, shaking, and stood outside the door, which I had left cracked open. I hear her moving, and after what feels like an eternity, I open the door.

"Mom, are you okay?" She stands in a pool of blood with her IV hanging loose. Blood everywhere—hospital gown and streaming down her arm and hand, on the floor. It looked like she tried to commit suicide. I lost it.

"Oh, my God! What have you done?" I screamed. Startled, she looked at me like a scolded little girl.

"You don't have to yell at me!" she cried.

I ran to her hospital bed, pushed the call button, shouting, "Please come help me! My mother has pulled out her IV and is bleeding like crazy."

"We will be right there," the nurse replies as Mom walks out of the bathroom, trailing blood.

"Mom, stay right where you are. The nurses are coming to help."

The nurses rushed in, calmed her, and stopped the bleeding. A nurse assistant begins to mop up the blood, and the other brings a wash pan of soapy water with a stack of towels and washcloths. My mom stands naked beside the bed on a towel while the assistant bathes her. She looks like a bag of bones. It's shocking!

"Let's move her into a room across from the nurse station and put in another IV," the nurse says to the assistants.

I stand in the room crying. My hands are shaking. I feel so horrible about screaming at her. I lost it instead of being the concerned daughter. I can't do this!

As they finished getting Mom back in bed with a fresh adult diaper and gown, I texted my sisters about what had happened. Shannan, the voice of reason, takes charge as she always does.

I think it's time to get Mom out of the hospital. No more IVs! She was picking at her IV all night long. She will just pull it out again. Let's bring her back to Memory Care. She texts.

Good idea. I will dress her and tell the nurse. I text.

Scott and I will come to get her and bring her back to Memory Care. Erin texts.

I tell the nurse we want them to release her, and she doesn't argue with me.

"I'll let the doctor know," she says.

I'm sure they can't wait to get us out of here.

I pulled out the clothes I found in her closet that morning: bright yellow pants, a pale-yellow cotton shirt, and a pretty yellow, black, and white floral pattern cardigan sweater.

"Mom, I'm so sorry I yelled at you. I love you."

"I love you too," she says quietly.

"Good news! We are taking you back to your apartment, and I brought you this cute outfit for you to wear."

"Oh, I forgot about this sweater. I love it!"

I help her dress. I brush her hair and wipe her face. I pulled out some lipstick from my purse and applied it to her lips.

"You look beautiful, Mom!" She smiles, and we hug.

The nurse comes in with release papers, and I sign them. She goes to get a wheelchair but doesn't return, and Mom is restless.

"Let's go," she tells me.

Miraculously, we hold hands and walk out of the room, past the nurse station, down the hall, into the elevator, and out the hospital's main entrance. She looks pretty in her pretty yellow floral outfit. She's smiling and has a spring in her step. She looks carefree. She is free from the bondage of the IV!

At the curb, Erin and Scott pull up.

"There you are! Look how cute you look, Mom," Erin says, gets out of the car, hugs Mom, and then helps her get in the front seat.

"We've got this. I called Memory Care, and they are waiting for us. Go home, Peg," Erin says. She can see in my eyes that I'm traumatized.

"Thank you. Bye, Mom. See you tomorrow." I say, choking back tears. Erin hugs me and gets in the car.

I watch them drive away. I feel like a total failure. There's nothing left for me to do but go home, and I drive in silence, my mind whirling.

I park the car under the carport, walk into the house, up the stairs, into our bedroom, and crawl under the covers, crying. The image of my mother bleeding everywhere burned in my mind.

Will this be the image I remember after she's gone? God help me.

I don't want my mom to suffer anymore. I know she hates living like this. This horrible disease is killing her. There is no hope for her recovery from Alzheimer's. My mother is dying, and I pray she won't suffer as she did the last 24 hours.

I must show her how much I love her during the limited time left. Will she forgive me for the outburst today? Will she even remember it?

I have been fighting her disease, but I can no longer resist the Big A. I am raising the white flag. I surrender.

CHAPTER SEVENTEEN
DON'T FORGET HOW GOOD
YOU ARE

It has been a week since my mom's hospital stay, and I am still running the horrific hospital scene repeatedly in my mind. It's like a bad movie: my raised voice, her hurt eyes, the way she looked like a scolded child. It haunts me day and night. I am ashamed. This is not how a loving daughter should react. How could I be so harsh when she was at her most vulnerable? If only I had spoken calmly and with compassion.

Memories of my mom nursing me from sickness keep surfacing. From getting my tonsils out as a child to having sinus surgery in college, she was always there. She had bedside manners that no one could match. If I had the flu or a virus, she'd set up a TV tray next to the sofa, bringing me chicken noodle soup, saltine crackers, 7-Up on crushed ice, and orange sherbet. She would kick Dad out of their bed at night, and I would curl up beside her.

In high school, I once had a high fever and remembered floating above my bed and looking down at the two of us from above. At that moment, I felt so much love for my mom, and I was back in my body within seconds. I'm not sure if it was a dream fueled by the fever or an actual out-of-body experience, but that feeling of being taken care of and loved so fiercely has stayed with me.

Later, living in Los Angeles, I had several surgeries. Mom insisted on flying out each time to be by my side. She spoiled me by cooking my favorite meals—Irish Stew, Red Beans and Rice, and Roast Beef with rice and gravy—and served them to me on a tray while I recovered on the sofa. We watched our favorite movies and shared laughter.

Once I was feeling better, Dad would drop us off at the nail salon for mani/pedis, followed by lunch at a neighborhood restaurant, Aroma Cafe, with the cutest garden! You ordered the most delicious salads and sandwiches at the counter, and they would bring them to your table. It was always packed, with everyone vying for the tables outside. Many times, we saw celebrities.

We even had small adventures: standing at Griffith Observatory, gazing from the Hollywood sign to the Pacific, or driving up the Pacific Coast Highway for a fabulous lunch at our favorite Malibu restaurant, Geoffrey's. Seated at the cliff's edge, looking down at the crashing waves, I ordered the ultimate California comfort food - Corn and Blue Crab bisque served with hot rosemary rolls fresh from the oven. Sunshine, ocean views, good food, my parents, and Jimmy sitting across the table were perfect and all I needed to feel better. I was blessed to have my parents with me as I recovered. My mom's laughter filled our condo and brought a smile to my face. Her magic touch and love were healing.

Growing up, my mom was never sick. If she got a cold, it would last a day or two and be over. Then in 2002, she was diagnosed with ovarian cancer. When she found out at the doctor's office, she grabbed her purse, said thank you, and walked out of the office. She went down two floors to my sister Kelly's office, told her the news, and then stood up to leave.

"Where are you going, Mom?" Kelly asked her.

"I'm going to get my nails and hair done," she declared, and off she went.

My mother believed everything would be fine, and it was. She had a hysterectomy the following week. She was lucky her cancer was only Stage I. She didn't need chemo or radiation, and her cancer never returned. She is a cancer survivor and believed she would always be cancer-free because she didn't dwell on it. She just knew she would be okay. She had too much living left to do. Her positive thinking carried her forward!

But positive thinking cannot cure Alzheimer's. It can only carry us through each hard day. Since I left the hospital last week, I have avoided going to see my mother at Memory Care. What if she remembers my outburst? What if she turns away from me?

Dad and my sisters have visited and reported she is a bit stronger and eating a "little." A bite? A sip of protein drink? A spoonful of yogurt? No one can really say.

"I need to go see Mom today. I feel ashamed I haven't gone to visit her." I tell Jimmy.

"I understand. Do you want me to go with you?" he asks. He knows how much I have been struggling.

"No, I will be okay."

"Okay" is my default. I'm lukewarm, half-alive. I feel like I have lost all passion for life. I smile because that is what we were taught to do.

When we were very young, Mom had a friend visit who tried to engage us in a conversation, but we were shy and didn't say anything. After the friend left, my mom sat us down and told us just to smile if we didn't have anything to say to her friends. The Sweeney smile was born. We all have big smiles and always take great pictures. We have trained our husbands how to smile for perfect family pictures, and the grandkids and even the great grandkids have all learned from example. They didn't have a choice.

My friend, Carmen, loves to tease us whenever we line up for pictures.

"Do the Sweeney smile!" she says to everyone else in the picture. She learned fast.

The Sweeney smile has helped me survive many uncomfortable situations and probably got me in trouble, too. Living in New York, I learned to curtail the smile after several strangers started following me on the street because I had innocently smiled at them. These days, it's my mask. If I smile, everything is okay, right?

My family loves pictures. We constantly annoy our husbands, kids, and friends by posing and snapping pictures. My parents' house is filled with framed photos, and the living room cabinets are stocked with countless photo albums. There are endless plastic bins of photos in their paper envelopes from the days we printed rolls of film. Most pictures have my mom's writing on the back of them. She would write a cute caption to accompany the photos with the place, date, and ages of everyone. She adored her photos and taught us to love them too. Taking pictures is a Sweeney family hobby!

For the last ten years, we have graduated to printed photo books. My sisters, Shannan and Kelly, are the queens of organizing them and creating beautiful hardback books for special occasions. Some of these photo books sit on my mom's nightstand at Memory Care. She used to spend hours looking at these at home, but now she only looks at them when one of us visits and opens the photo books to show her the pictures. She loses interest fast, and this puts another knife into our hearts. It is just one more thing that has changed. One more thing to remind us, she isn't the mother we knew. Add it to the lost list. The lost list gets longer, but we will never be able to check off "found." Those memories are lost forever. All the beautiful qualities of our mother have faded away.

My favorite photo book is the one from her 75th surprise birthday in New Orleans. It sits on the coffee table at home. We didn't bring this one to Memory Care. Maybe it will spark memories for Mom and for me. I grab it off the coffee table and walk out the door.

Driving across town, I pray. Please, God, give me the strength to get through this visit with Mom. Please let her be happy to see me. Please let her recognize me. Please help her eat. Please help her talk. Please don't let her die. We aren't ready. I'm not ready.

When I arrive, Mom's sitting with a group at a table. Deana, the Activities Coordinator, plays music on her cell phone, singing along to oldies but goodies. Some of the patients look amused, and some try to sing along. Deana stands and gives me a big hug.

"Hi, Mom. How are you today?" I smile, and she smiles back. She seems happy to see me. Maybe she has forgotten the hospital incident. I hope so!

Deana begins playing Whitney Houston's *I Will Always Love You.* It is one of Mom's favorite songs. I pull Mom up to her feet, and we dance while I sing to her. Well,

I dance. She just stands there, and I swing her arms and sing to her. The words of the song make me cry. I realize Mom isn't singing anymore, but she mouths the words, "I will always love you," and laughs weakly.

Deana grabs my phone and videotapes it. Mom gets tired quickly, and I sit her back down in her chair. Our dance lasted only about 30 seconds, but I will cherish the moment and the video. It is the dance of Alzheimer's, and I wonder if this will be the last time I dance with Mom.

Thanks, Deana," I say as she hands me the phone.

"You are going to want to keep that video," she says warmly, smiling at me.

The caregivers begin moving everyone into the dining room for dinner and place Mom in the kitchen area at a table. I follow and sit next to her.

"We are still monitoring her eating," Tiffany tells me.

"Good. Thank you."

I sat with her. I help feed her yogurt and hold a protein drink up to her mouth. She takes a few bites and a few sips. That is the best we can do today. She doesn't talk.

The caregivers buzz around Mom. They are wonderful, warm, and fuzzy. It brings me comfort.

"Mom, do you want to go to your room?"

She shakes her head, and I help her stand. We amble down the hall to her room. She sits in her wingback chair, and I show her the photos in the birthday picture book.

"Look, Mom, this is your 75th birthday. Remember when we surprised you at the hotel in New Orleans? I flip through the pages, and she looks at a few pages before staring away. I noticed she had written something on the back page of the photo book. I will bring it home and read it later. I lean it against my purse on the kitchenette counter and bustle around, organizing her outfits and straightening her drawers. The snacks we bought months ago are stale. I throw them out. At this point, she isn't going to eat them and probably would choke on them if she did. I grab a handful of the now stale Goldfish snacks—mindless Goldfish eating. I'm not even hungry, but I grab another handful.

The little solar-operated plastic red bird we bought at the Dollar Tree last year is sitting on her nightstand. It isn't getting enough light, so the wings are lifeless, just like my mom. I move it to the window, and in a few seconds, it begins flapping its wings.

"Look, Mom, your little red bird is trying to fly!"

She just looks at me. I remember how tickled she used to get when we had the bird on the windowsill of the kitchen. I feel like that bird, flapping my wings and going nowhere as I trudge my way through this visit. I'm not sure if she understands what I'm saying or what I'm talking about. It's painful. I turn on the TV, and *Jeopardy* is playing. She stares at the TV and taps the top of her mouth with her fingers. Heartbreaking. Fifteen minutes feels like two hours.

Crystal, the nurse, comes to give her the nightly meds. I watch as she crushes Mom's pills and mixes them into pudding in a small cup. She walks over, and Mom opens her mouth as she spoons the pudding into Mom's mouth.

"Swallow it, Miss Sherry," she says, and my mom closes her mouth and miraculously swallows it. *Good girl.*

The caregivers will soon be coming to prepare her for bed, and I will try to figure out my exit. I use her bathroom and notice a large box of adult diapers on the bathroom counter. Since the hospital stay, Mom has been wearing these now—a new constant. I can't imagine how humiliating it is for her, or maybe she thinks this is normal.

"Mom, I need to leave now. I have to fix dinner for Dad and Jimmy."

326

"Oh, you're leaving?"

She reaches for me to help her stand. It is the first thing she has said since I arrived, and she is alert for this moment. Life has come back to her.

We walked out of her room holding hands and go slowly down the hall. She stops at the sitting area halfway down the hall and wants to sit in the chair in the corner. She puts her legs on the hassock, lies her head back, and closes her eyes. She looks tired. My precious little mama is so small in this big armchair.

"Goodbye, Mom. I love you. I'll see you tomorrow," and I lean down to kiss her cheek.

"Bye," she says with her eyes still closed.

I turn to leave and then turn back to look at my mother again. Her eyes are now open, and she is staring intensely at me. At that moment, I feel like she is seeing me for the first time in years.

"Don't forget how good you are," she says.

"Thank you, Mama," I say, choking back tears.

She closes her eyes, and I turn and walk away, stunned.

Don't forget how good you are!

327

Those six precious words are what I desperately needed to hear today from my mother. Where did this come from? She has never said this to me before. These words of wisdom from my mom seemed to come from heaven above. It's as if God was telling her to tell me what I needed to hear to ease my pain. These words wiped out the movie in my mind of the hospital nightmare. This beautiful moment could be the new movie in my mind. I can replace it and will run it over and over again.

Don't forget how good you are. In these simple words, I know she has forgiven me and is trying to wash away my sadness.

Don't forget how good you are—the pat on my back I needed at this very moment. These words erase all regret, bad times, and sadness. I need to hold on to this.

My mother still loves me. She knows I have been with her and will stay with her until her last breath.

That night at dinner, I told Dad and Jimmy what happened and then shared Mom's words of wisdom. They smiled, knowing I needed the validation, Mom's words of encouragement.

After dinner, I pull out the birthday picture book to read the back inside cover filled with my mother's beautiful

328

handwriting. Dad sits with me in the living room, and I read it out loud.

This is my mother's story in her own words:

"Friday and Saturday, October 5 and 6, 2011,

My 75th birthday was a real surprise! Myles said he was taking me to New Orleans to stay in the French Quarter. We arrived at 3:00 p.m. and checked into our room. Myles went down to get us a cocktail. He returned and told me, "There is no cocktail service until later." We waited and watched a little TV and then went downstairs to the lounge. Still no drinks yet, so we talked with some guests sitting around us. I suggested we just walk around the French Quarter and buy drinks and snacks. There's a bar on every corner, right?

Myles then told me he had a business call to make and was gone for a little while, then came back and told me it was only thirty minutes before the Happy Hour began. He said the snacks were out, and we could help ourselves. He would be right back and left again. I started to get suspicious and wondered what was happening.

He returned with cheese and crackers, then asked me what I would like to drink. I told him a Bloody Mary. Then I saw him walking back with our drinks with a big smile. I smiled back and heard people singing "Happy Birthday to You" at the hotel entrance! My four daughters came to New Orleans to celebrate with us!

I was so surprised that I felt like laughing and crying at the same time. We had drinks and then walked to the French Quarter. We stopped and gambled for awhile at the Casino, then had a delicious dinner at Red Fish Grill. Afterwards, we went to Pat O'Brien's. The piano bar was too crowded, so we sat outside on the patio and had a great time together. We laughed, talked, and it couldn't have been any better, celebrating my birthday with my family, whom I love very much.

The next morning, we went for beignets at Café Du Monde for breakfast, then had a delicious late lunch at Commander's Palace before driving home to Baton Rouge. I appreciated all of my surprises. It will be a Birthday I will treasure, even though I turned 75!

Thank you to my precious husband for planning this surprise with my wonderful daughters. I am a very proud mother of all four of my girls. You are the best, and I love all of you so much. I hope we can do this again in the future. Love, hugs, and kisses, Mom."

Although we would never plan another surprise birthday weekend with just Mom, Dad, and my sisters, we can cherish the memories because we have a photo book filled with 140 pictures from the birthday weekend. Plus, we have my mom's beautiful story in the back of the book, describing how much the celebration meant to her and how much we meant to her.

As my mom's life winds down, what do I need to tell her before she is gone? I think I need to tell her how much I love her, and then I need to say, "Mom, don't forget how good you are!"

CHAPTER EIGHTEEN
EVERYTHING WILL BE
ALRIGHT

When did Friday night become just another night?

I remember when Friday nights were fun. I miss planning a date night or meeting friends for dinner or a movie. I miss going to hear live music. Friday plans are rare these days. When your mom is slipping away across town, you take it a day at a time.

I placed a frozen pizza into the oven, tossed a bagged Caesar salad, and set the table. I have no energy to meet friends or family, and neither does Dad or Jimmy. We are playing the waiting game, and Friday pizza is a good distraction. It doesn't even have to be a great pizza.

Pizza on a Friday night brings back childhood memories of going to Shakey's Pizza Parlor in Baton Rouge.

A small staircase led to a platform with a window overlooking the pizza makers. My little sisters and I would press our noses to the window, watching the dough fly in the air before the pies were shoved into the giant hot ovens. We loved our frosted mugs of root beer, sitting at long wooden tables with benches—way before community tables were a thing.

We often celebrated our birthdays there because they had a Dixieland band playing in the corner or a piano man playing ragtime. We'd gobble slices, then went home for birthday cake and Neapolitan ice cream. My sisters liked either chocolate or vanilla, but I wanted a scoop striped with all three flavors—just like my father. My mother liked the strawberry.

In college, I went to Fleur De Lis pizza with my theatre friends, usually after plays or rehearsals. We'd sit for hours—laughing, gossiping, flirting—pushing tables together to make one long table, sharing "Around the World Pizza," sipping cocktails or chugging cold pitchers of beer. The pizza was good, but the friendships were golden. Those were some of the happiest times in my life.

Later, in New York, while dating Jimmy, we would have Friday night pizza dates at Delizia Pizzeria on Second

Avenue. The hot garlic knots would melt in your mouth, and we would inhale them with an Italian salad. I would claim the banana peppers because Jimmy hated them. The pizza would arrive piping hot, with steam rising from the stainless-steel pan. I learned to fold my slice like Jimmy, careful not to scorch the top of my mouth. If we weren't too stuffed, we would share a sweet, decadent cannoli or a slice of spumoni and fight over the candied cherry on top until our friend, Roy, swore a candied cherry took 17 years to digest. After that, I let Jimmy have it.

Years later, flying into New York from Los Angeles at Christmas, Jimmy had our cab driver pull over at New Park Pizza in Queens. It was 11:30 p.m. I was tired from the long flight and ready to get to bed.

"Really, Jimmy? It is too late to eat pizza!" I snarled at him.

"I'm having pizza! Do you want a slice or not? I'm not sharing," he barked back at me.

"No," I said.

"Sir, do you want a slice?" he asked our cab driver.

"No. I'm good. Thank you."

Jimmy came back with two slices on a paper plate with napkins in a white bag, already bleeding oil.

"You got two slices?"

"Yeah!"

"Give me a bite!"

I took a bite. OMG! Best pizza ever! I didn't give it back.

"That's why I got two! I knew you would cave," he muttered, annoyed.

We chowed down our slices in the back of the cab on the way to his parents' house in Rockaway. That was the best slice of pizza I have ever had, and I almost missed it because I thought it was "too late."

A few years ago, I was in New York, meeting my friend Miriam to see a Broadway play while Jimmy met his best friend Kevin for dinner. I ducked into a stand-up counter pizza joint in the theatre district called Kiss My Slice. I loved the name, but the pizza was just okay. I still compare every slice to that freezing night in the back of the yellow cab with my Jimmy Dean.

It's never too late to eat pizza. Even frozen pizza can make you smile. Pizza changes your mindset, at least for a few minutes. Never pass up on a slice of New York pizza. There's nothing like it. It's the real deal!

I hear my dad's van pulling in the driveway. He opens the door, hobbles in, and pours a glass of wine. I pour sparkling water and add a slice of lemon, then sit at the counter on a barstool, waiting for the report. The daily news of Mom comes from my father, my sisters, or friends who have visited her. I listen and hug him.

There is no plan to fix it—just listen, be present, be. Then serve him a slice of pizza.

"How was Mom today?" I ask, knowing the answer, but it's part of our routine.

"Not good. She didn't even acknowledge me. She just stared ahead. I stayed for an hour, then left when they took her to the dining room for lunch," he says sadly.

"I'm so sorry, Dad. I'll go see her first thing in the morning."

I hate seeing my father like this as much as I hate seeing Mom waste away. She went from being angry at him for placing her in Memory Care to being nothing. I can see his heartbreak. His denial is gone. He finally accepts her

Alzheimer's and knows she has slipped away from him, from us.

This is the long goodbye. Dad seems lost because there is nothing he can do. My strong father—whose mission was to take care of Mom and his family—is now broken. His emotional pain weighs down his body; he can't stand up without groaning. Is it the pain from his knees, his heart, or one big ball of grief choking life out of him?

He can't even bring their favorite Wendy's Frosty chocolate milkshake to her anymore. The last few times he did, she barely took a sip. The milkshake melted in her refrigerator until one of us threw it away.

How much longer will this go on? It weighs on all of us—my sisters, the grandkids, and our friends.

The next morning, I forced myself to go for an early walk around the lake. The lake that calms me is a blur. The sun still shimmers, herons stand in stillness, geese glide, turtles sun on the logs—but my mind is across town with my mom. I can no longer appreciate the lessons of the lake. I can barely breathe. I'm lost in my thoughts, and before I knew it, I made a big circle and turned into our driveway.

I wash my face, brush my teeth, grab my purse, and head to Memory Care. I am still in my workout clothes, with no makeup, and my dirty hair pulled back in a hair clip. I find Mom in the main living room, sitting in a chair, and staring straight ahead.

"Hi, Mom. How are you?" I got no response.

"Are you hungry, Mom? Why don't we go to your room and get something to eat?"

No response. Nothing. She seems very weak. I helped her stand, and we walked to her room. I sit her in the armchair and grab yogurt and a small water from the fridge. I feed her a few bites, a few sips. She shakes her head.

"Do you want to lie down? I'm tired too, Mom. Let's lie down and take a nap."

Getting her into bed is a struggle. She grimaces and groans as I lift her legs to position her on the bed. It's not easy, but I finally settled her with a pillow under her head.

"Alexa, play Barbra Streisand music."

I hope this will comfort her. The music floats softly. I climbed in behind her, my arm around her waist. I listen to her breathing. Soon we breathe together. She feels so frail next to me. She falls asleep, and I hold my mother and cry and pray. *God, please take her to heaven. She would not want to live this way.*

The door opens, jolting me.

"Sherry Berry, do you need the bathroom?" a sweet caregiver asks. My mom suddenly woke up. She seems weaker than when I arrived. The caregiver helps her to the bathroom to change her. I hear Mom arguing with her, and I'm surprised. She has been so quiet all day. I get out of bed, drink bottled water and eat an apple I brought from home. They return, and she helps her back into bed.

Dad arrives at 2:00 pm. He sits in the armchair and watches her sleep. I grab my purse and sneak out. I drive home with silent tears. This just doesn't feel right. It feels like she is dying today.

"How'd it go?" Jimmy asks me from the back deck, cigar in hand. He just got home from golfing with our brothers-in-law. Golf with them is his saving grace. Cigars and golf keep him sane. I'm grateful for both. I am thoroughly checked out of this marriage right now. I have nothing to give. I have nothing to say.

I can't answer. He reads my face—despair, emptiness, and heartache—stands and hugs me.

"Twenty-two-second hug," he says, not asking. He knows I need it and probably much more.

"Are we still going out tonight?" he asks. We'd plan dinner and a movie.

"Dinner, but no movie. My mom is so weak. I'm worried about her. I want to check on her before we go to dinner. Is that okay?" I squeak out because the lump in my throat is so big I can barely speak.

"Sure, whatever you want to do," he replies, and I break from his comforting hug to go inside the house to shower.

I shower and cry under the hot water, blow-dry my hair half-heartedly, then crawl into bed for a nap. Emotionally hungover. Sleep is the only escape.

Jimmy comes into the bedroom and wakes me up a couple of hours later.

"Your Dad just got back. What time do you want to leave?" he asks.

"Let me get dressed and put some makeup on," I say.

You can at least make an effort, I tell myself. I drag myself out of bed and throw on white jeans, a cute top, and some sandals. I put on a little more makeup than usual—pink lipstick, earrings, and bracelets. I'm trying. Barely.

"Dad, how was Mom?"

"She slept almost the whole time I was there. I fell asleep in the chair. They came to get her for dinner, so I left," Dad says, defeated.

My dad looks so down, and I hate to leave him tonight.

"We are going to stop by Memory Care to check on Mom before we go to dinner," I tell him.

"Great. Thanks for doing that. You kids have a good dinner. I'll heat leftovers and read my book," Dad says.

My father is an avid reader, and the house is filled with books everywhere you look. I know his books are his refuge.

Jimmy and I silently walk down the path to the Memory Care entrance, sign in, and climb the stairs. Jimmy punches in the secret code, and the door swings open.

Nurse Crystal is in the hallway, and she tells me Mom took her meds but is weak from not eating. The kitchen staff shake their heads when I ask about dinner—sorrow in their eyes.

How do they endure this? They are my heroes. It takes extraordinary people to do this work. They deserve a place in heaven. They will always have a place in my heart.

We find Mom sleeping.

"Mom, I'm back. Jimmy's here." I say as we walk into her room. She opens her eyes, looks at me, and then closes them again.

Jimmy finds a baseball game on TV while I climb into bed and spoon Mom. My breath matches hers. She laces my hand with hers on her stomach. Now and then, I stroke her hair, face, and shoulder. I want to stay like this forever. I think I am comforting her, but really, I'm the one comforted by her touch, her breath, and her smell.

"I'm hungry. It's 8:15. Let's go. Tell your mom goodbye and meet me in the hall." Jimmy whispers as he stands up from the chair and leaves the room. His tone is cranky—low blood sugar—he needs to eat.

I crawl out of bed reluctantly. I don't want to leave.

"Mom, Jimmy is hungry. We are going to grab dinner. I will see you tomorrow. I love you."

"I love you," she says, opening her eyes to look at me.

I stand by her side, lean down, and kiss her. The light from the bathroom is the only glow. She then looks past me to the wall across from her bed. Chills run up my spine, and the hair on my arm lifts.

I'm back at my grandmother's deathbed—her fixed stare at the end of the bed, seeing her parents ready to take her home to heaven.

"Mom, what are you looking at?" I ask, not sure I want to know. Is it her mom, her dad, her brother? I feel someone there.

"I see Jesus' face. Mama has to go home now," she whispered, peaceful, eyes fixed on the wall.

I can't leave. My gut says this is her last night.

In the hallway, Jimmy waits.

"Jimmy, I can't leave her. I'm spending the night. She just told me she sees Jesus' face and Mama has to go home now," I say, crying but barely getting the words out.

"I don't understand what you are saying. Stop crying, so I can hear what you are saying," he says impatiently, but trying.

I breathe and tell him again, then slip back into the room and into bed with Mom, my arm around her waist. Jimmy comes back into the room and sits in the chair. I'm sobbing and holding onto Mom. She knows I'm crying as she can feel my shaking body pressed up to hers.

She starts to comfort me.

"It's okay. Everything will be alright. It's okay," she says, repeating as she pats my hand with hers.

Jimmy was watching us with tears falling down his face. After fifteen minutes, he kisses me.

"This is heartbreaking. Your mother is comforting you. Call me if you need me. I love you," he whispers to me.

After he leaves, the caregivers come into the room to change Mom. As they pull her nightgown over her head, she gets angry at them, she flails, throws her arms back, hits the wall, and slowly sinks to the floor. It is painful to watch. She is pitiful, and I feel helpless—as if life is seeping out of her and out of me.

Once they get her into bed, I pull a nightgown from her dresser and change into it. I tuck my contact lens in two small plastic medicine cups on the counter and find a new toothbrush in her bathroom drawer—my first overnight in Memory Care.

I barely sleep. I listen to her breathing, convinced each breath will be her last. One minute, we are entwined and breathing together, and the next moment, the caregivers enter the room to guide her to the bathroom.

Morning comes, and somehow, she seems better. The morning caregivers arrive and dress her for breakfast. As they walk her to the dining room, I change out of the nightgown and put my clothes on. My sisters and Dad are planning to visit Mom today. I'm exhausted mentally, emotionally, and physically. I want to go home, crawl into bed, and sleep all day.

Mom is sitting in the dining room with scrambled eggs and grits. A sweet caregiver is trying to get her to take a few bites.

"Goodbye, Mom. I love you," and I kiss her goodbye, leaving reluctantly.

Mama didn't go home to heaven last night, but she is ready—and it will be alright. I take comfort in knowing she is being watched over because she has seen Jesus' face. I believed her because she told me, and the look of peace on her face at that moment will be something I will never forget.

Cheese Grits Casserole

Ingredients:

4 cups of water
1 tsp. salt
½ tsp. pepper
1 cup of quick cooking grits
2 cups of shredded cheddar cheese
⅔ cup of whole milk
⅓ cup butter
1 tsp. Worcestershire sauce
1 tsp. garlic powder
4 large eggs, lightly beaten
Paprika to sprinkle on top

Instructions:

Bring the water and salt to boil in a large saucepan.
Stir in grits and return to boil.
Cover, reduce the heat, and simmer for 5 minutes, stirring occasionally.
Remove from heat and add cheese, milk, butter, Worcestershire sauce, and garlic powder.
Add eggs, stirring well.
Spoon mixture into a lightly greased 2-quart casserole dish.
Sprinkle the top with paprika.
Bake at 350°F for one hour or until lightly browned.
Let it stand for 5 minutes before serving.

Yield:

8 servings - You can double or triple for a buffet dinner.

Family Notes:

You can make this the day before and refrigerate it overnight. This recipe was always made by my brother-in-law, Robert Reiger's Aunt Shirley, for Christmas Eve. It is a great side dish for anything and perfect for brunch. It puffs up like a soufflé and melts in your mouth.

My easy version of cheese grits is to follow the quick cooking grits directions on the box, add a stick of butter and a small bag of shredded cheese, a few tablespoons of sour cream, and Creole seasoning.

I once brought a big crock pot full of easy grits to a church dinner in Los Angeles. A few people sneered at the grits. I overheard several say, "I don't like grits!" A few minutes later, everyone was raving about my grits and they all lined up fighting for the last spoonful. The minister asked me to email him the recipe so he could send it to everyone!

CHAPTER NINETEEN
THE LAST ANNIVERSARY

My beloved Mom has finally graduated from palliative care to hospice care. We're living with the dreaded reality that "the end is near." I'm not surprised, but this sucks. She can no longer walk and barely eats or talks. Five months in Memory Care, and she has declined so fast. Is it Alzheimer's, or has she simply given up? I know my mom would not want to live this way.

Last week, my dad went to visit her with Duncan, my 17-year-old nephew. As they were walking her back to her room, her legs collapsed beneath her. Hospice was called, and a wheelchair arrived within hours. Another symbol of surrender in the A-Zone.

"Mommee doesn't call me her boy anymore, and now she can't walk," Duncan told my sister, Kelly, that evening. He was devastated. Out of all the grandchildren,

Duncan is the one who visited her most consistently. He'd call my dad—Big Daddy to all the grandkids—to ask when he would be going and meet him at Memory Care. Dad was Duncan's strength and support, and Duncan was Dad's support during these visits. After visiting Mom, they would hit a local burger joint for lunch or dinner. It was their special Grandfather-Grandson bonding time.

Other days, Duncan would call Dad, ask if he could visit, and go fishing at the lake. Dad would walk out with him, sit on a bench, and watch him fish. He never catches anything, but it doesn't stop him from returning. I think fishing was just an excuse to hang out with Dad.

"Poor Duncan, he never catches any fish," Dad would say after he left.

"That's OK, Dad. I think he just really wants to hang out with you. You are lucky—most teenagers don't want to hang out with their grandparents!"

"You're right," he'd answer.

Lately, "you're right" is his refrain, a gentle surrender after years of Mom and his four strong daughters telling him what to do. It makes me stop and check myself: am I being too controlling? We all inherited that trait from our mom.

"Our 62nd anniversary is in two weeks," Dad announces.

"Oh, that's right. I forgot."

"Do you think I could take her out for a nice dinner? I want to get red roses for the table. Could you help me dress her in a nice outfit, put some makeup on, and fix her hair? I could take her in a wheelchair. I want it to be special—it looks like this will be our last anniversary."

"Dad, that is probably not a good idea, but I will discuss it with my sisters." Before I call them, Shannan texts:

We need to do something to celebrate Mom and Dad's 62nd Wedding Anniversary on June 22nd.

Dad wants to take her to a nice dinner, but I think that it's a crazy idea. I reply.

Yes, that will not work. We need to celebrate in Memory Care. Shannan texts back.

I will check to see if we can use the Community Room. Kelly texts.

Let's surprise both of them. Peg, maybe you can go early and make sure Mom has a nice outfit on? Erin texts.

It is hard to believe my parents have been married for 62 years. For better or worse, in sickness or in health. My parents are such a beautiful example of a long and loving marriage. My dad has honored his vows even though these brutal years with Alzheimer's have reshaped her into the woman he barely recognizes. His love remains. He just wants to have one more date night—one more lovely dinner—which can't happen. Heartbreaking, and somehow still inspiring.

They met when my mother was a freshman at Southeastern University in Hammond, Louisiana. Dad was with Frank Jackson, a friend he had grown up with in New Orleans. They both had attended LSU together. Frank was dating my mother's best friend, Margaret. The women won a college theatre contest and decided to spend their winning money on a girls' weekend in Biloxi, Mississippi.

Dad and Frank rolled up to Biloxi in Frank's convertible, surprising the women at the hotel bar with cocktails and music playing from the jukebox. Dad had too much to drink, and my mother thought he was obnoxious. She made a pretend name for herself and introduced another friend as her twin sister.

"You aren't twins," Dad said.

Mom shot back, "We are fraternal twins."

When she left for the ladies' room, Dad told Frank and Margaret, "I'm going to marry her one day." They laughed and told him her real name was Sherry Murphy.

"You lied to me, Sherry Murphy! Now you have to dance with me!" Dad said to her when she returned.

"There's no dance floor here. We can't dance on the carpet!" Mom exclaimed.

Dad pulled her up anyway. She laughed at him, and they danced on the carpet between the crowded tables. She led as she was the better dancer.

The next day, seven of them piled into the red-and-white Ford convertible and drove to Pensacola Beach. Mom sat on Dad's lap for the two-hour ride. Talk about a way to get to know someone. They were inseparable from that day on!

Dad had just accepted a sales job in Birmingham, Alabama, but every weekend he would drive back to Louisiana to see her. One night, they drove through City Park, and as they went around a traffic circle in the middle of the park, the Fats Domino's song, "I'm Walking," began playing on the radio. My dad pulled the car over to the side, cranked up the music, and they jumped out to dance in the circle. People drove by, honking their horns and clapping for them. They laughed, danced, and kissed under the moonlight. Dad knew this was the woman for him.

Mom was beautiful, fun, loved life, and him. Her mother's Cajun cooking didn't hurt. Soon, they were engaged, and my mother quit college after her first year to plan her wedding. She was only really attending college to get her MRS degree. She worked as a clerk at an insurance company to save for their wedding. She designed and made her wedding gown, as well as the flower girl's dress. They got married on June 22, 1957, at St. Alphonsus in the Irish Channel of New Orleans, with the reception at Lenfant's Hall, and honeymooned back at the Buena Vista Hotel in Biloxi, where they had first met.

Soon, they settled into a small apartment in Birmingham, Alabama, where I was born the following July. Later, they lived in Lafayette for a few years, then settled in Baton Rouge when I was five years old. Four daughters, four sons-in-law, and nine grandchildren, plus three step-grandchildren, their love has been the glue that holds the family together. Their love is worth celebrating!

Once we secured the Community Room at Memory Care, we went into full sister event-planning mode. We ordered a cake, sandwiches, chicken fingers, fruit, and chips.

Shannan booked the piano player, who occasionally sings at the assisted living unit. The party will just be our family, including the grandkids who live in Baton Rouge. We gather framed pictures of Mom and Dad to display, and Kelly frames a photo of their wedding invitation. Shannan asks me to find the wedding cake topper from their wedding cake. We remember seeing it in a glass dome with a wooden base, but it is nowhere to be found.

"Dad, we are planning something, so don't ask me any questions," I tell him. "I will meet you at Memory Care at 5:00 p.m. on Wednesday, and I will take Mom to her room to dress her in a nice outfit, brush her hair, and put some lipstick on her."

He wants his beautiful wife back. It breaks my heart to see how disturbed he is by Mom's disheveled appearance. In his mind, he believes that with the right outfit, hair, and make-up, she could be the Sherry he wants to remember— loving, vibrant, funny, full of light and laughter.

"That sounds great," he says, and I can see the hope flickering in his eyes—this will be a special anniversary even though he can't take her on a date.

I asked Jimmy to get some festive helium balloons and pick up the food I ordered. Erin is bringing champagne

354

and orange juice to make Mom her favorite mimosa. Everyone is excited to surprise them, especially with the piano player. We know Mom will love it!

Dad is already there when I arrive at Memory Care, sitting in a big armchair, shaking his head sadly. I see Mom slumped down in her wheelchair, expressionless. She seems feebler than before. The caregivers who know about the party have dressed her in a nice top and brushed her hair. It doesn't make sense to take her down to her room and try to redress her in her favorite pink jacket, which I brought from home. I whip out lipstick from my purse and dab it on her lips. She stares right through me. We are a few weeks late with this celebration.

"Mom, it's your wedding anniversary. We have a surprise planned for you and Dad," I say in the most upbeat tone with a smile on my face, swallowing back tears.

All set. I text my sisters.

We are ready! They replied.

Here we go. Dad and I wheel Mom out of Memory Care. As we enter the Community Room, we hear the piano player playing and singing "It's A Wonderful World," and we make our grand entrance. Everyone shouts, "Happy Anniversary," and then—just as quickly—faces fall.

None of us have seen Mom this frail. It's the worst the grandchildren have ever seen their beloved Mommee.

One by one, they all step forward to hug Mom and Dad, wishing them Happy Anniversary. As they step away, I hug them, and tears begin to roll. Mom doesn't acknowledge any of it. My mother, who loved celebrations, seemed oblivious to the anniversary party. Dad is impressed with the party, especially the music. He is grateful and thanks each of us for making this happen.

Erin raises the mimosa to Mom's lips—a tiny sip. We stood around eating sandwiches and fruit, pretending to enjoy the party. The piano player strikes up "New York, New York,"—our song! I walk over and stand in front of Mom, grabbing her hands and begin "dancing" with her and singing along. Whenever we heard this song, we would always jump up, do leg kicks, and act out the lyrics pretending to be Liza! Miraculously, at this moment, there is a flicker of recognition in her eyes. She smiles and perks up. She shakes her head to the music and moves forward, as if she wants to stand up.

"Dad, come dance with Mom," I shout to him across the room. He's startled. Everyone looks at me like I am crazy. Maybe I am. But we have to catch this moment, and

Mom clearly wants to dance. Dad and I help her stand up, and we hold her from each side with our arms around her waist as we begin swaying to the music. Another song begins. I step away so they can dance together, and for fifteen beautiful seconds, my parents dance and celebrate their 62 years of marriage. We stand around them crying.

Kelly captures the special moment on her Nikon. We settle Mom back in the wheelchair and try to keep the party going as the piano player continues to play more of her favorites.

She fades again, and we wheel her to the cake table. Shannan points out their framed wedding pictures and wedding invitation. Mom looks confused. We all sing "Happy Anniversary" to you in our most pretend—happy voices. Kelly cuts the cake. Plates passed.

I stand there stuffing cake into my mouth, not tasting a thing. The pain in the room is unbearable. I can barely breathe.

Erin feeds Mom a bite of cake; she holds it in her mouth, not chewing, not swallowing. I guess it will melt down her throat, I think. Erin goes to give her another bite, and she shakes her head. It hits me that this will be the last party, the last family celebration with our mother. There will

357

be no more Thanksgiving dinners, Christmas parties, Easter, or birthday celebrations with her.

How can we bear it? She was our rock, who taught us the art of celebrating as only a Southern mother can do. I could never live up to her "hostess with the mostess" touch and never tried.

I walk into the little kitchen attached to the community room and sob quietly. Jillian, my 13-year-old niece and the youngest granddaughter, sweetly walks over to hug me. We hold onto each other for several minutes. Her compassion touches me, and I will never forget that hug.

As an adult daughter, it is hard for me to accept Mom like this, but I can only imagine how difficult it must be for the grandchildren. I was an adult before I lost three of my grandparents and my aunt to cancer, but watching their wonderful grandmother, who they all adore, waste away from Alzheimer's has to be gut-wrenching for them.

Our fabulous music man plays one more song as we begin packing up the food, which barely has a dent. We cut a slice of cake for him and brought the rest to the kitchen of the Memory Care. None of us wanted to look at the anniversary cake again. The staff are grateful to have been a part of the celebration and gush over how wonderful it is that we had this party for Mom and Dad. They are excited to have a slice of the cake.

"Can I help Mommee back to her room?" my nephew Duncan asks me as I begin rolling the wheelchair out of the room.

"I can get that," Dad exclaims.

"Sure, that would be a great help, Duncan," I say as I give Dad a look.

I step aside, letting Mom's youngest grandson take the lead. Dad and I follow them, and Dad steps forward to punch in the security code to open the Memory Care doors. As they slowly open, I turn around and see my sisters and husbands carrying out the leftovers and champagne. Jimmy hurries up with the flowers to Mom's room. We left the balloons behind. The last anniversary party is over.

"Aunt Peggy, can you take a picture of Mommee and me?" Duncan asks as he stops in the living room area, handing me his phone. He rests his hands on her shoulders and bends down to kiss the top of her head. Mom tilts her head down as if blessed by his kiss. They stay like this for several seconds, still and entwined, gathering strength from each other. It takes my breath away. I think of the beautiful Pietà I saw at the Vatican many years ago—but here, it is a grandson, comforting his dying grandmother. This loving moment, captured on a cell phone, is an image I'll carry forever in my heart.

A caregiver follows us to Mom's room to prepare her for bed. Dad, Duncan, Jimmy, and I walk out into the night, down the path to our cars, stunned and quiet. Lost in our grief. We hug Duncan goodbye and drive home.

Back at the house, I set their framed wedding invitation and the black and white wedding picture on the bookshelf across from Dad's chair. They're so young in the picture, cutting their cake—smiles were full of hope and promise. And they delivered, a life of ups and downs, daughters, grandchildren, friends, beautiful homes, holidays, and travelled across the country and the world. The house is full of photos—memories of better times.

I hope when Dad looks at their wedding photo and invitation, he will remember the good times, the carpet dance at the Buena Vista, the moonlit dance in City Park, Mom walking up the aisle at St. Alphonsus church, and all the beautiful years of a well-lived life together when she was healthy, and her spirit was bright. I hope he holds tight to the love from 62 years of marriage with the woman of his dreams. And, when he looks at the grandchildren—and soon-to-be great-grandchildren—he will see Mom's spirit shining through and give him the strength to go on.

I hope my mother knew she was surrounded tonight by her precious family, who love her deeply, beyond words—who can't imagine life without her. May she stay with us and give us the strength to keep shining in this world without her.

Happy Anniversary, Mom and Dad! We love you! I love you!

CHAPTER TWENTY
A SHERRY SKY

"Do you want to go see the pandas at the National Zoo during lunch? It's always been on my bucket list to see them," my sister Shannan asked as we grabbed a coffee and a muffin from the back of a large meeting room before settling in for a three-hour workshop.

We both served as alum advisors for our college sorority and had come to the convention in Washington, D.C., with our group of LSU girls. After four long days of meetings and banquets, we were desperate for fresh air.

"Sure, that sounds great. I've always wanted to see the National Zoo," I replied.

Half an hour later, Shannan noticed a text on her phone and stepped quickly out of the room, looking worried, and motioned for me to stay put. I pulled out my phone and saw the sisters' group text from Kelly:

Mom is now on oxygen, and hospice has ordered a hospital bed for her room. Call me.

My stomach dropped. I hustled out of the room and found Shannan on her phone. I could hear Kelly filling her in. Mom had taken a sudden turn for the worse.

Our flights weren't until the following afternoon. It was July 1st, right before the Fourth of July—changing a ticket would be nearly impossible.

"Let's finish the workshop, and we can talk at lunch," Shannan said. We both held back tears, trying to focus on the presentation, but our minds were spinning.

The truth is, I'd had a bad feeling before we even left Baton Rouge. The day before we left, as I walked out of Memory Care, I thought: *What if this was the last time I saw Mom? Maybe we shouldn't go.*

But after talking it through with Dad and my sisters, we decided to stick with the plan. We made the commitment months ago. The sorority girls needed two alum reps to attend the convention with them. Plus, Shannan's daughter, Caroline, was having a wedding shower in D.C. on Saturday night, and we were planning to attend. Life was still happening as my mom's life was slipping away. Hospice told us it could be weeks, even months. Mom might be rallying as she did before.

After the workshop, we changed into casual clothes and walked a mile to the zoo. It was a beautiful summer day. On the way in, I grabbed a hot dog from a cart, and for a moment, I felt like I was back in Central Park.

We made our way to the Panda Sanctuary, edging through the crowds until finally—there they were. The famous Pandas. Except, they were fast asleep, sprawled across rocks behind glass. It was disappointing and uneventful, but we saw them.

"I can scratch that off my bucket list," Shannan sighed. Her dream of seeing the Panda family frolicking in their sanctuary was dashed.

Her phone rang as we walked up the path to the main entrance. It was Kelly on FaceTime.

"I think y'all need to change your tickets and come home ASAP. Mom may not make it through the night," she told us in her direct doctor's voice. She then flipped the camera. We saw Mom lying in a new hospital bed, unresponsive. My niece, Mackenzie, stood on the side of the bed and held up her baby, Tripp, for Mom to meet for the first time. My mother, the "baby whisperer," didn't move, didn't even blink. It was shocking. Dad, Kelly, and Erin were standing around her deathbed while we were standing in a zoo watching helplessly through a phone screen. It was unreal.

Seriously, God? After this suffering—this is how it ends? We won't even be there to tell her goodbye. It felt like a nightmare.

We looked at each other, holding back tears, turned, and walked briskly out of the zoo. Back at the hotel, Shannan called the airline. At first, they quoted $600 each to change the flights. Through tears, she explained the situation. Miraculously, after holding for ten minutes, the agent returned: the fees would be waived if we could make the 5:30 p.m. flight. Within an hour, we were packed and waiting for my niece Caroline to drive us to the airport.

How do you breathe knowing your mom is probably dying? The lump in my throat was strangling me, but there was nothing to do but pray and hope we would make it back in time to say our goodbyes.

The flight home was the longest of my life. I prayed non-stop:

Please, God, let us make it in time to tell Mom goodbye. Please don't let her die before we get there.

365

When we landed in New Orleans, Kelly texted:

Mom's oxygen level is dropping. Hurry!

Rob, Shannan's husband, was waiting at the airport curb. He threw our bags in the back of the car and sped us to Baton Rouge. I continued to pray in the backseat for the hour drive to Baton Rouge. The sun was setting as we drove. The sky turned a brilliant pink.

"Look, Shannan, the sky is pink," I said, breaking the silence in the car.

"Nanny is here to take Mom home," Shannan said.

We both remembered the pink sky the night our grandmother died. The Pink Nanny sky was back.

"The heavens are opening up for Mom," I said, and we both started crying.

Rob dropped us off at the front door, and we ran into the Memory Care—up the stairs, punching in the security code, through the automatic swinging doors, past the caregivers in the kitchen, past the nurse giving out meds to the residents, and down the hall. It felt like slow motion, and we would never arrive. I finally made it through the door into the room with Shannan following right behind, and our mother was still alive—a miracle.

The room was crowded: Dad, Jimmy, my sisters, three brothers-in-law, my nephew Duncan, and some caregivers. Empty wine bottles and trays of food hinted at the all-day vigil. In the middle of it all, Mom lay in a hospital bed, oxygen tube in her nose, unresponsive.

I'm not sure if she knew we were here. Her eyes were half open, but she was just staring ahead. Erin and Kelly moved away.

"Mom, it's Peggy and Shannan. We're here, Mom. We love you, Mom," we told her gently, taking our places on either side of her.

The caregivers hugged her goodbye, "Bye, Sherry Berry. We love you," before heading off shift, tears in their eyes.

How lucky we were to have loving caregivers take such good care of our mother.

My sisters and I sat on the sides of the single hospital bed, crying over Mom, telling her how much we loved her.

"It's okay to go, Mama. Go to the light. We will be alright. We will take care of Dad. We love you, Mama," we told her repeatedly. But my mom didn't want to go. She was holding on.

I pulled out my cell phone and began playing her favorite music: Barbra Streisand songs: "Memory," "The Way We Were," "People." Then, YouTube videos from *The Sound of Music*. We sang along to "My Favorite Things," "Edelweiss, and "Climb Every Mountain." And finally, "Sherry" by Frankie Valli.

Dad just sat in the armchair next to her bed, looking lost. Now and then, he reached over and touched her hand.

"I'm so glad you were able to get back," he told Shannan and me.

At midnight, only the immediate family remained.

"I think we should play soft piano music and turn out the lights. Let's get quiet. Maybe if we stop crying, Mom will be able to let go," I said.

"I guess we are all spending the night?" Shannan asked.

"I'm not leaving," I stated.

"Me either," Erin replied.

"It's a slumber party," Kelly said sadly.

"I guess I'm staying, too," Dad said.

Everyone was exhausted. The crying had stopped. At this moment, we had no more tears to shed.

Shannan, Erin, and Kelly climbed into Mom's double bed, which had been pushed against the wall to make room for her single hospital bed. Dad sat in the wing-back chair, closing his eyes.

I played soft piano music on her Alexa, turned off all the lights except the bathroom light, and climbed into the hospital bed with Mom. She was lying in the middle of the bed, with maybe six inches left on the side for me. I lay on my right hip, teetering on the edge of the bed, with my left leg balancing on top of my right leg. It was not an ideal sleeping position. My left arm draped over her chest, and my fingers were on her neck so I could feel each breath. Her breathing was shallow, but it wasn't the horrible death rattle I remembered my grandmother had when she was dying.

"We haven't all slept in the same room since camping in the pop-up camper," Shannan joked, and we all laughed, remembering the good ole days.

The beautiful, calming music settled us down. Soon, everyone was asleep. I could hear my dad snoring.

"I love you, Mama. It's okay to go now," I whispered in her ear. I didn't feel tired, but somehow, I drifted to sleep.

The next thing I knew, I was falling in slow motion. I hit the floor with a thud.

The room stirred awake.

Erin popped up, "Are you okay?"

"What happened?" Shannan blurted out.

I was on the floor trying to pull myself up in a stupor. My hip hurt. My arm hurt.

"Peggy, turn the light on!" Dad said.

I finally pulled myself onto my knees and tried to turn the lamp on, but it was dark, I was half awake, and I couldn't find the switch. I fumbled for a few seconds before finally turning the light on.

"Is she still breathing?" Erin said as we stared at Mom.

"Yes, she is," I replied.

We fell silent, watching our mother. Within seconds, we heard her take her final breath, and then I said the dreaded words:

"I think she is gone."

Our beloved Mama was free. She was out of pain and no longer suffering from Alzheimer's. She was whole again as she moved into the next realm. I know in my heart that her mother, father, and brother were there to bring her to heaven. She was now our angel.

The next hour there was a blur. We stepped out of the room while the caregivers dressed her in a clean nightgown with her pretty pink robe. They crossed her hands, smoothed her hair, and she looked peaceful.

The wonderful executive director of the Memory Care facility showed up even though it was now 2:00 a.m. We took turns kissing Mom and telling her we loved her, then let Dad spend some time alone with her.

At 2:30, the hospice representative arrived and announced her time of death.

We sat in the waiting area, discussing the last minute of her life. Thank God I had fallen off the bed, waking us all up! It would have been awful to have a caregiver come in and wake us up to inform us that our mom had passed.

It was strange and beautiful. We all believed that our grandmother's spirit or Mom pushed me off the bed to wake us up.

"Wake up, you don't want to miss this moment!" Nanny was saying.

Or Mom, "Get with the program, move on, enough of this crying."

There was nothing else for us to do. We were drained of tears and exhausted. We all went home to get some sleep. We would talk in the morning.

I always imagined that when I lost my mom, I would be in the fetal position on the floor in the corner of my room, crying hysterically, unable to move, but that was not the case. We went home. I hugged Dad goodnight and went to bed at 3:30 a.m.

The next morning brought phone calls, arrangements, and tasks. The funeral home staff was compassionate and gentle. My mother would be cremated, and we would have a Memorial Mass on July 16th.

When we returned to Mom's room, most of her furniture had already been moved out by the brothers-in-law. I packed her clothes into plastic bags to drop off at Goodwill. Before leaving, I grabbed her little red plastic solar bird we had bought at The Dollar Tree and stuck it in my purse. We said goodbye to the staff, thanking them for the loving care of our mother, then dropped the keys to Mom's room at the front desk. Our time here was over.

Walking out of Memory Care that was Mom's home for just over five months, seemed so final, and I cried as I walked down the path to my car. I was grateful for the excellent care she received, but I found freedom in knowing that we wouldn't have to come here anymore to witness her cruel fate of Alzheimer's.

Back home, I placed the little red bird on our kitchen windowsill, and soon, the wings began flapping in the sunlight. There was something comforting about that little red bird. I've heard that when you see a Cardinal, your deceased loved ones are telling you they are thinking of you. From now on, every Cardinal will be Mom.

Two days later, Dad and I met with Father Uter, our childhood parish priest, who agreed to say her Mass at the Cathedral. Years ago, he had renewed my parents' vows for their 50th Anniversary. Mom loved him and would be pleased. We also rented out the parish hall for the reception following the Mass.

I planned to write a tribute to my mother, but I procrastinated for days before finally sitting down to write it. Surprisingly, it flowed freely, and I felt her presence guiding me. In my heart, I knew she would be proud of me and love every word.

On Friday, July 16th, we celebrated my mother's life. The church was packed with family and friends. We framed the beautiful picture I took of Mom standing in front of the pink azaleas and set it on an easel to the left of the altar. Our family friends, Pierre and Angelle, sang "Ave Maria" and a few more of Mom's favorite songs. My nephews and my niece told stories of their beloved grandmother, Mommee. They were sweet, funny, and touching. I followed them, and I felt Mom's presence as I stepped up to the podium. I spoke about her love and her life, and these are the last two paragraphs:

"A month before Mom passed, I was visiting her, and when I was leaving, she looked at me and said, 'Don't forget how good you are!" These words would be the last wisdom I would receive from Mom, but I believe they were for everyone who knew her. Mom was an amazing wife, mother, grandmother, aunt, cousin, mother-in-law, and friend—but remember, you are amazing too, because you opened your heart and let her in. You let my mom teach you about life. You let her be your cheerleader. You let her teach you how to be a friend.

So, whenever you look up and see the sky turning pink, please know in your heart that it's a Sherry Sky—her way of reminding you not to forget how good you are!"

After the funeral, everyone walked to the parish hall to continue celebrating her life. The room resembled a wedding reception—flowers everywhere, "food for days" spread across a long table in the center of the room, with a huge dessert table off to the side. Hundreds of pictures of happier and healthier times played on a large screen, along with her favorite music. People laughed, hugged, kissed, and shared stories of Mom. It was joyous and exactly how my mother would have wanted it.

"Mom, this party is for you," I thought, looking around at all the beautiful people who adored my mother—the cherished ones she had loved so much.

"Peggy, I must tell you something. Your mother was with you on the altar," my mom's dear friend, Miss Pat Delage, told me at the reception.

"I know I felt her, Miss Pat."

"When you were giving your mom's tribute, the sun was streaming through the stained-glass windows and filled the back wall of the altar with pink light. It was perfect—it gave me chills," she exclaimed.

"Thank you, Miss Pat. I needed to hear that," I replied, hugging her close.

"I've never seen anything quite like this for a funeral. Your mother was truly loved," the church secretary told me as we carried the extra food and flowers to our car,

"Yes, she was!"

Two days later, the sky turned brilliant pink at dusk, and family and friends who saw it began texting us. They sent pictures they snapped from their porches and backyards. Dr. April, my mother's doctor and friend, posted her pink-sky photos on Facebook, tagging my sisters and me.

"It's a Sherry sky! We will never look at a pink sky again without thinking of your beautiful mom."

EPILOGUE

The enlarged picture of my mother in her bright pink jacket, standing in our backyard in front of the beautiful blooming azalea bushes, sits on a table in our foyer. I walk by it many times throughout the day, and it warms my heart. Sometimes, I stop and look into her eyes and whisper, "I love you, Mom. We miss you!"

Grief is the great leveler. None of us can escape it. But it can also guide us—teaching us how to live more abundantly. I'm no longer afraid of grief, because it shaped me into the woman I am today.

A few nights ago, I saw a beautiful Downy Woodpecker perched on a street sign. His black, white, and red feathers shone in the light. I'd never seen one before and wondered if this was another lesson. Curious, I looked up the spiritual meaning: creativity, optimism, and the courage to follow one's desires. It also symbolizes protection, communication, and the ability to uncover hidden truths.

The woodpecker's persistent drumming can symbolize persistence, rhythm, and divine timing in life. That bird carried the exact message I needed in this season of my life—six years after my mother's passing.

Life can change in an instant.

Embrace the timing

Every minute, the good and the bad.

Look for the pink cloud moments.

They are everywhere.

Even in the darkest days,

They can lift you up and remind you...

Don't forget how good you are!

And don't forget to eat the pie!

RESOURCES FOR CAREGIVERS

Books
- *Pink Cloud Moments: A Sacred Space Journal for Caregivers* by Peggy Sweeney-McDonald
- *The 36-Hour Day* by Nancy L. Mace and Peter V. Rabins
- *Loving Someone Who Has Dementia* by Pauline Boss
- *Creating Moments of Joy* by Jolene Brackey
- *How to Sit & Stay with Compassionate Meditation* by Sabrina Johnson
- *Being Mortal* by Atul Gawande
- *Finding Meaning: The Sixth Stage of Grief* by David Kessler
- *Learning to Speak Alzheimer's* by Joanne Koenig Coste

Podcasts
- *Life in the A-Zone* with Peggy Sweeney-McDonald
- *Fading Memories* with Jennifer Fink
- *Daughterhood the Podcast*
- *The Alzheimer's Podcast*
- *Help for Alzheimer's Family and Spouse Caregivers*
- *Alzheimer's Speaks* with Lori La Bey
- *Soul Pathology* with Amanda Rieger Green
- *Listen In, Listen Up* with Sabrina Johnson
- *All About Alzheimer's* (Alzheimer's Foundation of America)
- *Remember Me* (personal stories about dementia)
- *InsideWink* with Jean Trebek and Allison Martin

Organizations
- *Women's Alzheimer's Movement* — womensalzheimermovement.org
- *Alzheimer's Association* — alz.org

- *Alzheimer's Services of the Capital Area* (Baton Rouge) — alzbr.org
- *National Institute on Aging* — nia.nih.gov
- *Family Caregiver Alliance* — caregiver.org
- *AARP Caregiving Resource Center* — aarp.org/caregiving
- *Hilarity for Charity* — wearehfc.org
- *GriefShare* — griefshare.org

Speaking Engagements & Workshops

Peggy Sweeney-McDonald is available for speaking engagements, book events, journal workshops and caregiver support programs inspired by *Life in the A-Zone* and *Pink Cloud Moments™*. Peggy shares her bittersweet caregiving journey and creative path through uplifting talks and workshops for caregiver support groups, churches and community organizations.

For speaking inquiries, please email:
PinkCloudMoments@gmail.com or visit
www.PeggySweeneyMcDonald.com

CAREGIVING TIPS

If you are on the caregiving journey, please take care of yourself. These tips may help:

- **Begin and end your day with stillness.** Pray, meditate, or simply take five minutes to breathe. Guided meditations on YouTube are great, especially if you struggle to fall asleep.

- **Keep a gratitude journal.** Write down at least three things every day—small joys add up. Write down your wins and challenges each day.

- **Find a support group.** Look for groups through your local Alzheimer's services, caregiver or grief groups through local churches.

- **Make the tough decisions.** Your loved one may want to stay in control but remember—they are no longer capable of making safe decisions.

- **Move your body.** Get sunshine, take a walk, or try yoga or exercise videos on YouTube (5, 10, or 30 minutes).

- **Bring in music and laughter.** Play songs, dance, or watch shows that incorporate music. Laughter counts as medicine—watch a comedy, a comic show, or even cat videos.

- **Eat to fuel, not just to cope.** Stress makes sugar and alcohol tempting, so stock up on healthy alternatives like fruit, vegetables, nuts, dark chocolate, yogurt, and herbal teas. Take multi-vitamins.

- **Ask for help.** You don't have to do it all.

- **Talk to someone.** Find a therapist or a trusted friend who will give you a safe space to vent.

- **Practice self-compassion:** Write a letter praising yourself for the good things you're doing. Let go of guilt, hold on to grace. Look in the mirror and smile, you are a hero.

- **Accept the sacred and the messy.** This journey isn't perfect—it's challenging, but full of grace.

- **Find beauty in the ordinary.** Those little moments are your *pink cloud moments.*

- **Grab a coloring book.** For you and your loved one, coloring is relaxing, creative, and an excellent way to connect. Sit side by side, pick up some crayons or markers, and color away—it's a simple meditation you can share together.

- **Dream ahead.** Watch travel videos on YouTube and imagine the vacation you'll take one day.

- **Remember, you are not alone.** There is a whole community walking this path with you.

ACKNOWLEDGEMENTS

Writing this book has been the most healing journey of my life. I could not have walked through the A-Zone without the love, support, and encouragement of so many people.

To my beloved father, Myles Sweeney, and my sisters—Shannan, Erin, and Kelly—thank you for walking this challenging road by my side. We carried each other through Mom's Alzheimer's journey, and I am forever grateful for your love and strength.

To my husband, Jimmy, my best friend and anchor—you gave me grace on the days when I had nothing left to give. I need your 22-second hugs always, even on the days I think I'm okay.

To my nieces and nephews, who keep me young and bring so much joy to our lives.

For Stephanie, for suggesting the girls' weekend with our mothers—memories for a lifetime.

For Anne, Janet, Fran, Jennifer, Melanie, and Missy—my oldest friends who are still cheering me on.

To Natalie—closest to a daughter I'll ever have—who makes me smile and gave us Benji.

To Jackie Begue and Katherine Martin—thank you for bringing your creative hearts to my *Pink Cloud Moments* journals and standing with me in this next season of storytelling.

For Pennie and Sherry, my writer friends who encourage me to keep showing up to the page.

To Alice, my spiritual coach and prayer warrior, who keeps me on the path.

For Kathryn, the first person I told about my idea for the Caregiver Journal, and she said YES.

For Michel, my Los Angeles BFF, who moved to Baton Rouge and is now my soul sister.

For Nancy, who taught me how to record the podcasts in a closet over Zoom, and for the laughs.

For my Sunday Sisters, who hold my hand and show up with grace, support, and vulnerability.

To Maxine, Alice, and Karen, who befriended me at a crawfish boil and became my dear friends.

For Sabrina, who encourages, inspires and supports me from Arizona.

For Carmen, who makes me laugh and tells me to do the Sweeney Smile!

To the staff at Sunrise Memory Care—thank you for treating my mother with love and dignity.

To my extended family and dear friends who listened, comforted, and reminded me to laugh—I love you all.

ABOUT THE AUTHOR

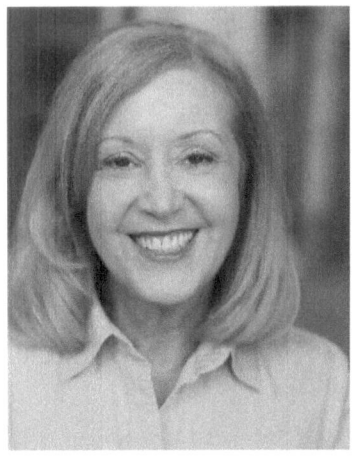

Peggy Sweeney-McDonald is a Southern storyteller, actress, and author who believes in the power of memory, food, and family to connect us all. Raised in Baton Rouge, Louisiana, and a proud graduate of Louisiana State University. She has spent her life weaving heartfelt stories into books, journals, a podcast, theatre and live events.

Her memoir, *Life in the A-Zone*, grew out of her bittersweet caregiving journey with her beloved mother, Sherry, and her popular podcast of the same name, which has been downloaded in over 30 countries. She is also the creator of the **Pink Cloud Moments™ Journals**, including the *Pink Cloud Moments - A Sacred Space Journal for Caregivers* and the *Pink Cloud Moments Divine Angelic Inspiration - A Sacred Guided Journal*, designed to bring comfort, joy, reflection, and creativity to those walking through grief, caregiving, change, and personal transformation.

Peggy's earlier work includes creating and producing the live food monologue show *Meanwhile, Back at Café Du Monde… Life Stories About Food*, which toured nationwide and was published as a book by Pelican Publishing. She continues to explore new creative projects, including *Pink Cloud Moments in Paris*, a travel memoir; *Voodoo Princess*, a young adult fantasy novel; and additional works that celebrate resilience, creativity, and magic in everyday life.

Peggy has been a presenter at the **Louisiana Book Festival**, **The Faulkner Society Words and Music Festival**, and **Empowered Women**. She was honored at **A Celebration of Women**.

Her writing has appeared in M*edium, InsideWink, Chili Pepper Magazine, InRegister Magazine*, and *Thrive Global*. She was featured in *Bluffs and Bayous, 225 Magazine, The Advocate, California Caregiver,* and *The Arrow Magazine.*

She has appeared on both stage and screen, winning Best Featured Actress for her portrayal of Amanda in *The Glass Menagerie* and later acclaimed for her performance as Della in *The Cake* at Theatre Baton Rouge. She played Melissa in *Love Letters* at the Old Governors' Mansion for Valentine's Day. She was nominated for Best Actress at the Storer Boone Awards in New Orleans for her performance of Miss Alma in *Summer and Smoke.* She is a long-time member of Screen Actors Guild-American Federation of Television and Radio Artists (SAG-AFTRA).

Peggy lives in Louisiana with her husband, Jimmy, and her 90-year-old father, Myles. She loves traveling abroad with her husband, father, and family—always on the lookout for the perfect meal, croissant, gelato, museum, cathedral, concert, park, or magical experience. She continues to inspire others to "look for the pink cloud moments."

Learn more at peggysweeneymcdonald.com or lifeinthea-zone.com

ALSO BY PEGGY SWEENEY-MCDONALD

Pink Cloud Moments™ A Sacred Space Journal for Caregivers
A guided journal offering comfort, reflection, and creative space for those walking the caregiving journey with inspiration from the *Life in the A-Zone* podcast and memoir, writing prompts, caregiving tips, and resources.

Pink Cloud Moments™ Divine Angelic Inspiration Journal - A Sacred Guided Journal
A journal inspired by angelic artwork by Katherine Martin, featuring prose, messages of encouragement, writing prompts, and coloring pages designed to bring peace, hope, and spiritual guidance.

Meanwhile, Back at Café Du Monde... Life Stories About Food **by Pelican Publishing**
Based on the presentations of *Meanwhile, Back at Café Du Monde...*, these sixty-seven food monologues invoke your own special comfort food, recalling tasty memories of life, love, family, and friends to warm your heart, feed your soul, and make you pause to savor the sweetness of life!

Life in the A-Zone **Podcast on Apple Podcast, Spotify, Pandora, and other podcast platforms.**
A heartfelt podcast where Peggy shares her bittersweet caregiving journey with her mother, Sherry, blending love, laughter, life, and loss. Downloaded in over 30 countries, these episodes offer comfort, connection, hope, and "pink cloud moments" to listeners walking their own caregiving paths.